MONITC
THE CRIT
ILL PA1

Patient Problems
and
Nursing Care

MONITORING THE CRITICALLY ILL PATIENT

Patient Problems
and
Nursing Care

Carole Rainbow
RGN, Dip.N (Lond.)

Senior Sister, Intensive Therapy Unit,
Bristol Royal Infirmary

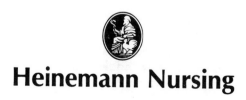

Heinemann Nursing

Heinemann Nursing
An imprint of Heinemann Professional Publishing Ltd
Halley Court, Jordan Hill, Oxford OX2 8EJ

OXFORD LONDON SINGAPORE NAIROBI IBADAN
KINGSTON

First published 1989

British Library Cataloguing in Publication Data

Rainbow, Carole
    Monitoring the Critically Ill Patient
    1. Medicine. Nursing
    I. Title   II. Series
    610.73

ISBN 0 433 00084 8

Photoset by Wilmaset, Birkenhead, Wirral
Printed in Great Britain by Biddles Ltd
Guildford and King's Lynn

Contents

Preface

Monitoring techniques previously reserved for use in the operating theatre are extending into other areas of the hospital. In addition, in those areas of the hospital such as intensive therapy units, more frequent and more invasive monitoring techniques are becoming commonplace. This leads to a number of problems.

Nurses who are unfamiliar with the technique in use may well be unhappy with either the practical or theoretical management, and an unhappy nurse is not tuned in to the patient.

The problem of lack of theoretical and practical knowledge also produces the twin spectres of a patient's decline (and demise) being beautifully documented but not acted upon, or alternatively artefactual readings being accepted as gospel. This is a difficulty not only with nursing staff but also with many junior medical staff who will either ignore or act inappropriately on information which they do not understand.

This book should go some way towards redressing the balance and could be read to good effect by either of the above groups although it is obviously aimed at nursing staff in high dependency areas.

Bob Winter MRCP, FFARCS
Clinical Research Fellow

Acknowledgements

For my mother and father.

I would also like to acknowledge the tremendous help and encouragement given to me by Jenny and Andy Lolley. This includes the assistance with illustrations, typing, helpful criticism and advice, as well as the provision of regular nutrition.

My grateful thanks.

Carole Rainbow

1

The Electrocardiogram

INTRODUCTION

The use of sophisticated equipment within the ward setting is an anxiety provoking experience for both patient and nurse. This chapter deals with the practical aspects of the most common monitoring procedure encountered, ECG (electro-cardiographic) monitoring.

In the same way that it is not vital to understand the internal workings of the telephone in order to make a call, it is not important for a nurse to understand the internal workings of the ECG machine in order to take a recording and interpret it. However it is essential to know how to use an ECG machine. Using this analogy it can be seen that, to make a phone call dialing the correct number is essential, though without lifting the receiver it is useless. Likewise, correct connection to the ECG monitor is desirable but useless if the operator cannot find the power button to turn the machine on!

In addition to the equipment, it is important to acquire a good working knowledge of the organ concerned, the heart. It is a complex mechanism but not too difficult to understand.

A further important consideration is coping with the profusion of technical words and jargon that the subject is laden with. Some important 'do's and don'ts' for the nurse to bear in mind are:

1 Don't be put off.
2 Don't use jargon yourself.
3 Do understand the meaning of technical terms and be able to explain them in a simple way.

Electrocardiography

Electrocardiography literally means a graph or trace of the electrical activity of the cardiac muscle. To begin with we must first consider the anatomy and physiology of the heart and the properties of the cardiac muscle.

THE HEART

The heart is the pumping mechanism of the body. It maintains the circulation of the blood to the tissues and ensures that the oxygen, nutrient, and waste disposal needs of these tissues are met. The **left and right sides** of the heart are **separate**, although they **contract together synchronously.**

The left side of the heart receives oxygenated blood from the lungs via the pulmonary veins, which it discharges into the arterial network of blood vessels via the aorta. The right side of the heart deals with deoxygenated blood from the superior and inferior vena cavae, which it discharges into the lungs via the pulmonary artery. The atria act as reservoirs of blood, supplying the main pumping mechanisms of the heart, the ventricles. Valves situated at the border between atria and ventricles prevent regurgitation, or reverse flow of blood into the atria. They are called the **mitral** or **bicuspid** valve on the left side of the heart, and the **tricuspid** valve on the right. The atria contract simultaneously, followed shortly afterwards by synchronous ventricular contraction.

ELECTRICAL CONDUCTION MECHANISM OF THE HEART

In normal physiology there is a defined conduction pathway. This pathway begins with the specialized group of cells termed the sino-atrial node. As its name suggests, the sino-atrial node (SA node), is situated in the right atrium. It has the highest intrinsic rate of all the tissues in the heart, at approximately 80 beats per minute, and is termed the pacemaker.

The SA node initiates an electrical activity which passes rapidly through the atrial muscle. This electrical activity is relayed through the second specialized area of conducting tissue, the atrio ventricular node.

This node is situated at the junction between the atrial and ventricular tissue. The wave of electrical activity is passed through the node and down a bundle of conducting fibres, the Bundle of His, which is located in the ventricular septum.

The atrio-ventricular node (AV node), can initiate its own contraction waves at a speed of approximately 60 beats per minute, which is slower than the SA node. The Bundle of His subdivides into left and right bundle branches within the ventricular septum. Each of these bundles serves a ventricle, then further subdivides to form a fine network of conduction tissue, or fibres, which infiltrate the ventricular muscle. These fibres, termed Purkinje fibres, also have the ability to initiate contraction waves, but their intrinsic rate is only 40 beats per minute.

You will have noticed that at certain points in the heart, the cells can begin their own electrical activity, but this is usually much slower than that initiated by the SA node. If such an event occurred, the waveform would be different in shape because of the abnormal route it must take to travel around the heart.

Electrical stimulation of the muscle cells is brought about by changes in the ion concentrations within the cell and in the surrounding extracellular fluid. At rest, the electrical charge within the cell, measured in millivolts (mV), is -70 mV. At the initiation of a contraction, sodium ions (Na^+) in the extracellular fluid move into the cell, causing a change in the electrical charge. During this change, potassium ions (K^+) escape from the cell into the extracellular fluid. Gradually more Na^+ ions enter the cell raising the electrical charge until it becomes less negative. When the voltage reaches -60 mV, it is deemed to have reached the threshold. At this stage the cell is committed to an all-or-nothing response, i.e. to contract, or not to contract.

The continued 'leakage' of Na^+ ions into the cell increases rapidly to a point were the electrical charge within the cell becomes $+30$ mV. Displayed on a graph this would show as a spike. This is termed the action or depolarization spike.

The cell must now return to its resting phase to prepare itself for the conduction of the next contraction phase. This recovery phase involves removal of the Na^+ ions from the cell, by the sodium pump, and retrieval of K^+ ions from the extracellular fluid. This process of recovery is termed repolarization.

Following repolarization there is a short pause before the next depolarization. The sequence of depolarization and repolarization takes approximately 0.8 seconds. This is termed the cardiac cycle, which is composed of ventricular systole, 0.3 seconds, and ventricular diastole, 0.5 seconds. Any increase in heart rate causes shortening of diastole, which means less recovery time for the heart between contractions.

Although the heart has four chambers, electrically they act as two. The atria have little muscle and therefore the resulting electrical charge is small. However, the ventricular muscle mass is large, especially within the left ventricle, so consequently a much larger amount of electrical activity is involved in ventricular contraction. The cardiac muscle fibres are collectively termed the **myocardium**.

Atrial activity as seen on the electrocardiogram (ECG) is usually confined to a small sized wave at the beginning of each set of complexes. This is termed the P wave. Ventricular activity is more easily seen and is of a larger configuration, it is termed the QRS complex, and follows the P wave. The T wave follows the QRS complex, it is the return to the resting, or repolarization phase of the ventricular muscle.

When recording the ECG, a baseline must be established. This is seen as a straight line on the recording to which the pen always returns called the isoelectric line. (See Figure 1.1). Movements of the pen or stylus either upwards or downwards are termed deflections. Upward movements above the isoelectric line are termed positive deflections and downward movements are termed negative deflections.

LEADS AND ELECTRODES

An electrode is a form of sensor. The electrode is the means by which a recording of the electrical activity of the heart can be 'picked up' through the skin. It may comprise of a small

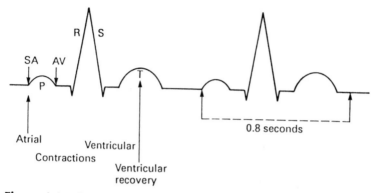

Figure 1.1 *Demonstrates the sequence of events occurring during the passage of the electrical impulse through the heart tissue.*

adhesive pad or a metal plate. Each of these is primed with a salt based jelly which improves contact with the skin. It is important to note that correct positioning of electrodes is vital if misinterpretation of the resulting trace is to be avoided.

In general terms the combined wave of contraction through the heart is downwards and towards the left side of the body. By placing electrodes near the left side of the body the heart's electrical activity on contraction will spread towards those electrodes, with the resulting deflection being positive, i.e. above the isoelectric line. If electrodes are placed so that the electrical activity or current will be moving away from them, there will be a negative deflection. (See Figure 1.2).

When observing heart rhythm it may only be necessary to use two electrodes, however a third electrode is added as an earth, this blocks out other artificial electrical interference from machinery which may be present at the bedside. If, however, a comprehensive three dimensional view of cardiac activity is required then a twelve lead ECG will be taken. The leads effectively look at the heart from twelve different positions, in either a vertical or horizontal plane.

THE TWELVE LEAD ECG

The twelve lead ECG is composed of six limb leads which look at the heart in a vertical plane, and the remaining six chest leads, which look at the heart in the horizontal plane.

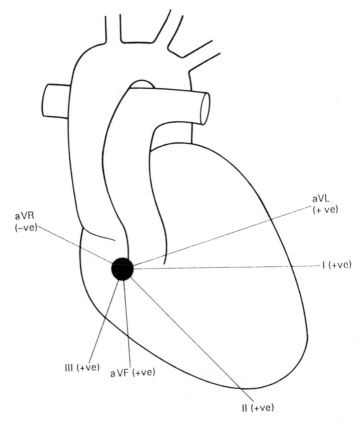

Figure 1.2 *The diagram demonstrates the position of the standard leads and the principle deflection recorded on the ECG (+ve upwards, −ve downwards).*

The six limb leads are coded as I, II, III, aVR, aVL, aVF:
- Leads I, II, and aVL look at the left lateral surface of the heart.
- Leads III, and aVF look at the inferior surface.
- Lead aVR looks at the atria.

As previously mentioned, the electrical current of the heart is downwards and to the left, this means that of the six limb leads, aVR produces a negative deflection on the ECG trace. When viewed on a paper trace aVR therefore appears upside down, the rest of the leads being mostly upright.

The chest leads are labelled V1 through to V6: Leads V1 and

V2 look in the direction of the right ventricle, leads V3 and V4 at the ventricular septum and V5 and V6 look at the left ventricle. (See Figure 1.3).

Electrodes used in ECG recording are of two types, unipolar and bipolar. The chest leads are unipolar in that the electrical activity recorded by the ECG machine is that which is detected by a single electrode, as it is placed in different positions on the chest. The limb leads are however bipolar meaning that the waveform displayed is the sum of the electrical activity detected by two of the leads.

MONITORING ECG

In most cases, ECG monitors have three main lead settings for continuous monitoring of heart rhythms. Leads I, II, III. Correct positioning of electrodes is vital if the nurse is to obtain an adequate trace with minimal distortion.

Objectives

Ensuring minimal patient anxiety while obtaining the best trace size and signal voltage for optimal observation. It is the rhythm and rate we are most interested in when observing with three lead continuous monitoring.

Equipment

- ECG monitor
- Electrodes x 3, (pre-gelled and disposable)
- Scissors, for clipping chest hair
- Alcohol pads

Procedure

Explain fully, in language the patient can understand, what you intend to do and why. Obtain the patient's verbal consent to being monitored, if they are able to give it.

1 Prepare equipment, turn on oscilloscope.
2 Apply ECG electrodes to prepared skin sites, correct application of electrodes will ensure a clear trace.

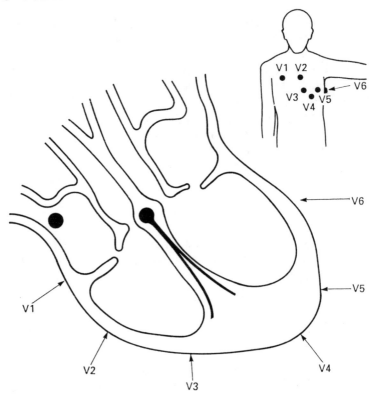

Figure 1.3   *Diagram denoting the position of chest leads.*

a Choose sites for electrode placement.
   Rationale: Care should be taken not to use areas of skin overlying skeletal muscle, e.g. lower end of the thorax, as movements of the ribs during respiration will cause interference on the waveform
b Clip chest hair around the area chosen for electrode placement.
   Rationale: Removal of hair improves conductivity and minimizes patient discomfort.
c Clean areas with alcohol pad, allow to dry.
   Rationale: Removal of natural oils from skin improves conductivity.
d Apply gel coated electrodes to skin sites, gently.
   Rationale: Pressure on the centre of the electrodes may

cause movement of gel onto adhesive, thus reducing skin contract.

3 Connect the electrodes to ECG monitor
- Red—Negative Lead
- Yellow—Positive Lead
- Black—Earth Lead

4 Select lead on monitor, either I, II, or III:
Lead II
The waveform displayed from Lead II, gives the best view of the cardiac muscle, as the lead looks closely at the apex of the heart. The electrical current passes down the ventricular bundles close to the position of Lead II. As a result the waveform is positive and of a large size, which makes interpretation easier. This is therefore the lead of choice for rhythm and rate monitoring. (See Figure 1.4).

5 Examine trace
a Ensure good quality of pattern.
b The R wave should be twice the height of the whole QRS complex to ensure correct ECG pickup by the alarm detector.

6 Set rate alarms.
The alarms must be switched on as there is not much point monitoring the ECG if dysrhythmia or monitor dysfunction is not noticed and remedied! As will be seen in Chapter 9, no one can continuously concentrate on the monitor screen and successfully recognize all dysrhythmias as they occur. The alarms are excellent servants which never get tired or lose concentration, providing they are set properly.

RELATED NURSING CARE

Ensure emergency resuscitation equipment is functioning and nearby. Monitoring the ECG is useless if potentially life threatening dysrhythmias cannot be treated promptly by resuscitative measures. Ensure safety guidelines are followed. The manufacturers of monitoring equipment supply the necessary safety information in the instruction manual. Medical engineering departments of most hospitals will check the equipment at regular intervals. Nursing staff should acquaint

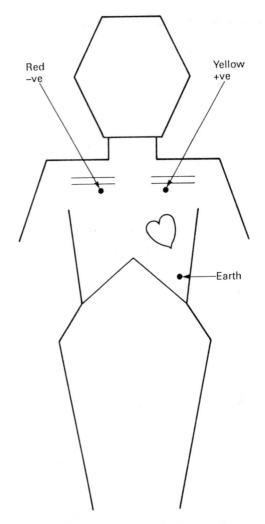

Figure 1.4 *Electrode placement to obtain lead II trace.*

themselves with the safety instructions when using all pieces of equipment.

In order to avoid interference or distortion of the trace, the nurse should prevent tension or dragging of lead wires, and check that electrodes are in contact with the skin and correctly connected to the monitor.

Use the monitoring equipment as a tool, but remember it

must be used in conjunction with observation of the patient's clinical signs. If an electrode, for example, falls off, the result will be a straight line trace on the monitor which would normally indicate asystole, the absence of any cardiac electrical activity. If the patient is breathing, of normal colour, and has a pulse, then we may conclude that he has not suffered a cardiac arrest and do not need to initiate resuscitation. The monitoring equipment must always remain a tool for the nurse to use, but should never take over our patient care.

Troubleshooting

1 Ensure the electrodes contain sufficient gel – insufficient gel on the electrode may cause a poor quality trace leading to artefacts (extraneous deflections). If the patient is cold and shivering, or just moving about on the bed, similar interference may occur. It is important to distinguish this from the clinical condition of atrial fibrillation which gives a similar picture on the trace.
2 Change electrode pads frequently. Rotate sites of placement and observe for signs of allergy and sensitivity. Use hypo-allergenic electrode pads if necessary.
3 Check for potential source of false alarm triggering.
   a High rate false alarm may be due to:
   - Muscle movement and artefacts.
   - Insufficient alarm setting above patient's own rate.
   - High gain setting, which may cause T waves to be counted in addition to the R wave thus doubling the rate.
   b Low rate false alarm may be due to:
   - Low gain setting.
   - Insufficient alarm setting below patients own rate.
   - Reduced R wave on a particular lead due to shift in the cardiac axis, see page 16.
   - Muscle artefact.
   c Other causes:
   Patient movement, loose or damaged lead connection, dry electrode pad, damaged ECG cable.
The continual sounding of alarms will be very frightening for the patient and reassurance that it is only a false alarm may do little to allay his anxieties.

Complications of Continual ECG Monitoring

1 Increased patient anxiety.
2 Damage to the patient's skin.
3 Equipment malfunction leading to incorrect interpretation.
4 Over reliance, by nurses on monitoring equipment.
5 Reduction in nurse patient contact.

TWELVE LEAD ECG

Objective

To give accurate data regarding the patient's electrical cardiac activity in such a way as to permit the diagnosis of a variety of important conditions such as myocardial infarction, myocardial ischaemia or ventricular hypertrophy.

Equipment

- ECG recorder, either single or three channel.
- Sufficient recording paper.
- Four limb electrode plates and straps.
- Chest suction cup electrode for single channel recorder.
- Six chest suction cup electrodes for three channel recorder.
- Electrode gel.
- Alcohol prep pads.

Procedure

1 Explain the procedure to the patient using language they can understand. Try to explain the reasons for taking the recording, thinking of yourself in the patient's situation.
2 Ensure privacy and warmth.
3 Position patient supine with arms, chest and lower portion of legs exposed.
4 Apply limb leads:
   a Use one electrode plate for each arm and leg. Although usually applied to the ankle and wrist, they may be applied further up the limb if necessary, i.e. post amputation.
   b Clean skin with an alcohol pad, allow to dry.
   Rationale: Removal of natural oils from skin facilitates good conduction and improves skin contact.

c Apply electrode gel to skin.
d Secure electrode plate straps to each limb.
  Rationale: Straps that are too tight are not only painful, they also increase any artefact on the reading.
e Attach limb lead cable wires to appropriate electrode plates.
  N.B. Each lead is labelled by colour and/or code to denote its position, e.g. LA refers to left arm, RA refers to right arm, etc.
f Check that each limb electrode is positioned properly and is secured to the appropriate limb.
5 Apply chest leads:
  N.B. Avoid draping the cable to the recorder across the patient's abdomen as this will cause artefacts due to respiratory movements.

Types of Recorder

Single Channel Recorder

1 Attach suction cup electrode to lead marked C.
2 Cleanse sites marked in diagram with alcohol pad and allow to dry.
3 Apply a small amount of gel to lead sites:
  V1: Fourth intercostal space, right sternal border
  V2: Fourth intercostal space, left sternal border.
  V3: Midway point between V2 and V4, left side of chest.
  V4: Fifth intercostal space, mid clavicular line, left side of chest.
  V5: Fifth intercostal space, anterior axillary line, left side of chest.
  V6: Fifth intercostal space, mid axillary line.

Three Channel Recorder

Attach all six suction cups to prepared sites at the same time.

Recording the ECG

Single Channel

1 Turn the lead select to STD, and centre the stylus.
2 Press the STD ImV button and adjust the machine to obtain

a needle deflection of 10 mm, (two large squares). This means that an electrical potential of ImV will produce a deflection of the needle by two large squares. The ECG recorder is then correctly calibrated and the variations in complex size can be correctly interpreted in terms of varying amounts of electrical activity rather than changes in the machine setting.

3 Check the paper speed is set at 25 mm per second.

4 Turn the select button to lead 1, record three or four complexes.

5 Mark the paper with the code 'Lead 1'.

6 Progress through all the leads i.e. Lead 1—Lead aVF, ensuring that the paper is marked with each lead code.

7 Switch to V setting, chest leads.

8 Record all chest leads by:

  a Placing the suction cup on V1—V6 sites progressively.

  b Turn the power switch to on, record three or four complexes at each site, marking the paper with the appropriate code at each setting.

  c Take a longer recording of the V1 lead; this rhythm strip, approximately 10 complexes, allows interpretation of the cardiac rhythm.

  d In moving from one chest position to another, ensure that the electrode is taken completely off the chest each time and then reapplied. If it is inadvertently slid over the surface of the skin to the next position, it leaves behind a trail of electrode gel which will conduct electricity. This means that the electrical current recorded in the new position represents the whole area covered by the gel not the single point where the electrode is in contact with the skin.

  e Finally, mark the paper with the date, time and patient name. Without this information the recording is useless.

Three Channel Recorder

1 Position all leads including the six chest leads before the recording is started.

2 Press the ImV button and adjust as necessary.

3 Depress the auto-run button, the machine will do the rest!

4 Label ECG recording with patient details, date and time of recording.

In the case of both types of recorder, the following is done:
1 Turn off the recorder.
2 Remove electrodes, clean gel from skin, ensure patient comfort.
3 Clean equipment.

Precaution

Ensure accuracy of lead placement to avoid misinterpretation of resulting trace.

Related Care

Assess twelve lead ECG for signs of dysrhythmia and intervene as necessary.

INTERPRETATION OF THE ECG

It is advantageous to adopt a logical approach to the interpretation of the ECG. This will ensure that potentially harmful dysrhythmias are quickly identified and treated. As we have seen the methods of recording ECG's are standardized. A knowledge of the position of electrodes and leads and the normal wave pattern viewed from these positions will assist the nurse to distinguish the normal from the abnormal.
1 Sinus Rhythm
The first thing to determine is whether the heart is beating in a normal sinus rhythm, i.e. is it under the control of the sino-atrial node. It will be recalled that the electrical activity in the atria associated with the SA node discharge appears as the P wave on the ECG. It is a matter therefore of checking to see if P waves are present and if they are followed by the QRS complexes associated with ventricular contraction.
2 Calculating Heart Rate
The next step is to calculate the rate. There are many approximate methods that can be used to assess heart rate

from the ECG trace. These depend however on the heart rate being regular. Two examples are given below:

a Count the number of QRS complexes in a three second period, (this is equivalent to 15 large squares), and multiply the result by 20.

b Count the number of large squares that occur between two consecutive R waves, then divide this number into 300, for example 300 divided by three (large squares) equals 100, the heart rate.

3 Is the Rate Regular?

A simple method to assess this is as follows:

a Lay the ECG flat, place a plain sheet of paper on the top or bottom half of the trace.

b Mark the position of an R wave on the plain paper, mark the following two R waves in sequence in the same way.

c Now move the plain sheet by one complex to the left, if the rhythm is regular the marks on the plain sheet will correspond to the R wave on the ECG trace. If the marks do not coincide with the R waves, the rhythm is irregular.

INTERPRETING CHANGES IN ECG CONFIGURATIONS

Aside from considering the changes that occur in the rhythm of the heart, which will be dealt with in the next chapter, there are changes that occur to the size, shape and pattern of the ECG complexes, which can indicate serious cardiac pathology.

Cardiac Axis

The mean direction of the contraction wave is downwards and towards the left side of the chest, this is termed the cardiac axis.

In the first instance it is worthwhile checking through the recording to assess whether the depolarization wave (QRS complex) is correctly depicted on the trace. Lead II is normally a positive lead, i.e. the QRS complex should be upright, but if this appeared as negative, (inverted) and if the recording is accurate, then this would indicate that the axis of the heart, has moved away from the normal position.

Changes in the axis are usually caused by disease processes. There are exceptions however, one of these being the rare case of dextrocardia, in which the heart is transposed to the right side of the chest. The most common cause of axis shift however is hypertrophy of the myocardium.

To view the normal axis look at leads I, II and III. All these leads should be positive, the largest positive deflection being seen in lead II.

Right axis deviation is usually caused by hypertrophy of the right ventricle. In this condition lead III will have a greater positive deflection than that of leads I and II, reflecting the extra electrical activity due to the enlarged ventricle on the right side of the heart.

Left axis deviation is caused by left ventricular hypertrophy. The enlarged left ventricle causes the cardiac axis to shift to the left as there is more electrical activity on the left side of the heart. Lead II therefore has a reduced positive deflection though it is only considered significant when this deflection becomes negative and inverted.

P Waves

P waves occur as a result of atrial contraction. As the atria contain little muscle mass the magnitude of the electrical P wave is small. On the ECG the P wave can have only two significant abnormalities, that is to say, they can lose their rounded shape and appear either pointed or notched. The pointed shape is due to right atrial hypertrophy, tricuspid stenosis or pulmonary hypertension. The notched or bifid shape is due to left atrial hypertrophy or mitral stenosis.

P-R Interval

Following the P wave there is a short pause on the ECG, this is termed the P-R interval. It is the delay during which the electrical current spreads down to the ventricles through the AV node. The normal range of time this process takes is 0.12–0.2 seconds, (three to five small squares). If the P-R interval is very short, it usually means that the initiation of the wave of contraction did not start at the SA node but further down in the atria. If the P-R interval is prolonged it may indicate abnormal conduction of the impulse from the atria to the ventricles. This situation will be dealt with further in Chapter 3.

QRS Complex

Damage to the conduction pathways prolongs the spread of the contraction wave through the ventricles, and is indicated by a wide QRS complex on the ECG recording, (i.e. greater than five small squares).

Q Waves

The first downward deflection on the ECG before the R wave is termed a Q wave. This deflection is not always present on the ECG. It corresponds to the first spread of electrical activity through the ventricular septum, usually away from the ECG electrode, hence the negative deflection. The significance of this wave depends on its size and where it appears on the trace. The Q wave does not normally appear as it is lost in the next phase of ventricular electrical activity which is a strong current through the ventricular myocardium towards the electrode, producing a large deflection upwards (R wave). If the Q wave is smaller than two small squares in height, depth or width, it is of no significance. If however, it is larger than two small squares, and is not present in leads aVR and Lead I, it is then pathological. Pathological Q waves appear on the ECG following myocardial tissue death. This effect can be understood if we consider the healthy ventricular myocardium which normally 'swamps' the Q wave with its own electrical activity. If the myocardium is infarcted, there will be no electrical activity as it is dead tissue, consequently the full Q wave will be visible. The infarcted area of myocardium acts as an 'electrical window'. Once pathological Q waves have appeared on an ECG they are a permanent feature and therefore while they indicate myocardial death they give no indication as to when the infarction took place. See Figure 1.5.

1 Early spread of electrical activity
   in intraventricular septum
2 Later spread in left ventricular
   myocardium, normally swamps 1
3 Area of dead myocardium acting
   as 'electrical window' due to
   absence of electrical activity as in 2

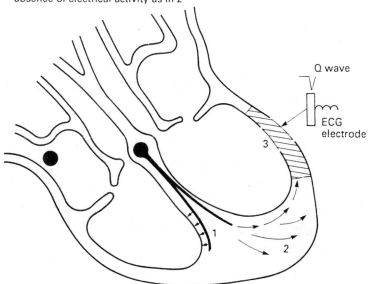

Figure 1.5   *Pathological Waves.*

R Waves

Changes in the shape of the R wave may be due to hypertrophy of the myocardium causing the R wave to be diminished in size. Posterior myocardial infarction may cause the R wave to become very tall.

S-T Segment

This portion of the complex, has a sharply defined outline, which is on the same level as the isoelectric line. If the segment is raised, it indicates damage to myocardial tissue by acute infarction or pericarditis. The damaged cells may be thought of as leaking positively charged potassium ions, hence the positive deviation from the isoelectric line. The leads that this abnormality appears in will indicate the site of injury, although in the case of pericarditis all the leads will be affected. An example of this would be if an elevated ST segment was seen in II, III and aVR. This would indicate an acute inferior myocardial infarction. See Figure 1.6. Depression of the S-T segment may be attributed to a number of conditions. For example, primary myocardial ischaemia appears as a horizontal depression of the segment with T wave remaining upright, but hypokalaemia and digitalis toxicity can cause an apparent sagging of the S-T segment.

T Wave

The T wave is usually a positive deflection and represents ventricular repolarization. The T wave is affected by electrolyte balance, giving rise to 'tall tented T waves' in hyperkalaemia, or increase in length in hypokalaemia. Inversion of the T wave is normally seen in leads aVR and V1, as these are negative leads. Some hours after a myocardial infarction, the T wave may become inverted due to myocardial ischaemia which is a common cause of inversion. Changes in the conduction pathway through the ventricles may also cause inversion of the T wave, particularly if the bundle branches are blocked. Ventricular hypertrophy is the fourth major cause of T wave inversion.

When reviewing the ECG it is important to follow a few simple guidelines

1 Is the heart rate regular?
2 Are P waves present, regular in rate, and the usual shape?
3 Is the P-R interval within the usual range?
4 Are significant Q waves present?
5 Are the QRS complexes the usual shape, height and width?
6 Is the S-T segment the correct shape, depressed or raised?
7 Is the T wave the correct shape, upright or inverted?
8 Is the axis correct?

ELECTROCARDIOGRAM — EXERCISES

1 What is the normal conduction pathway of the heart?
2 Where is the pacemaker and what is its intrinsic rate?

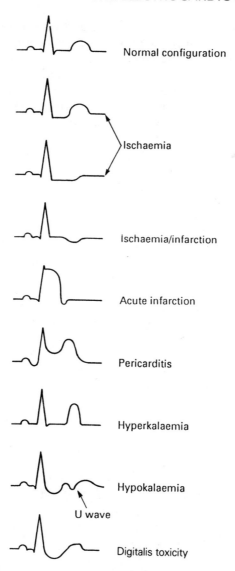

Figure 1.6   *Variations of the ST segment.*

3 How would you recognize a pathological Q wave and what are the causes of it?
4 How would you recognize left or right axis deviation and what are the causes of it?

5 What is the PR interval in time and what does it signify?
6 What is the normal length of the QRS complex?
7 What causes a raised ST segment?
8 What factors cause T wave depression?
9 How long in time is the cardiac cycle?
10 If there are five large squares between two consecutive R waves on the ECG what is the rate?

2

Common Dysrhythmias

Cardiac arrythmias may be classified into two major categories:
a Disorders of pacemaker function and impulse formation,
b Disorders of impulse conduction.
In this chapter we will deal with the former disorders, while the latter, known as heart blocks will be dealt with in Chapter 3.

It is important for the nurse to follow a thorough plan of action when interpreting the ECG, this prevents mistakes and ensures correct and prompt treatment of dysrhythmias. The guidelines in the previous chapter will help to establish such a routine. To keep matters as simple as possible, the heart will be divided into two parts, the supraventricular part i.e. everything above the ventricles, and the ventricular part. When discussing changes within the ECG recording it is worthwhile first learning the normal sequence of events.

SINUS RHYTHM

Sinus rhythm denotes normal electrical impulse formation and conduction through the heart. The rhythm is regular and the heart rate is 70–120 beats per minute. P waves, which signify atrial electrical activity, are present and regular in rate. The P-R interval is within the normal range, three to five small squares. Small non-pathological Q waves may be present in leads aVR and V1. QRS complexes are regular in rate and follow each P wave.

SINUS BRADYCARDIA

The impulse originates in the SA node and conduction is through the usual pathways. The rate of this rhythm is slow

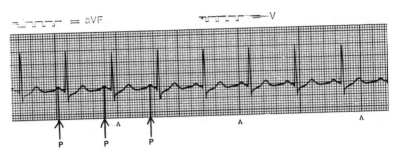

Figure 2.1 *Sinus rhythm.*

e.g. less than 60 beats per minute, and may be as low as 40 beats per minute. The P waves, P-R interval and QRS complexes are regular in rate and shape and appear in the correct sequence. This condition is not always significant. It may be present in young athletic types whose rigorous exercise programmes improve the efficiency of the cardiovascular system to the extent of reducing the heart's workload and subsequent rate. However certain disease processes do cause bradycardia, these include, hypoxia, hypothermia, myxoedema (hypothyroidism) and myocardial infarction.

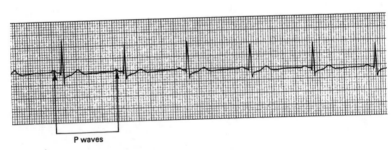

Figure 2.2 *Sinus bradycardia.*

The clinical significance of the rhythm is allied to its effects on cardiac output. Reduction in cardiac output gives rise to signs of shock and reduced tissue perfusion. When signs of reduced cardiac output are present the patient, may complain of angina, due to decreased coronary blood flow. Syncope, (fainting) and heart failure are also features of this rhythm.

It is possible for more serious dysrhythmias to develop as a result of bradycardia, this is particularly so if it appears as a symptom of myocardial infarction. Bradycardia need only be treated if symptoms are present.

NURSING INTERVENTIONS FOR PATIENTS WITH REDUCED CARDIAC OUTPUT

Assessment of the patient will reveal reduced cardiac output and symptoms of shock with associated reduction in tissue perfusion.

a The patient will need to be placed flat in bed, unless dyspnoeic.
   Rationale: This is to ensure that cerebral blood flow is maintained.

b Give prescribed drug therapy e.g. Atropine 0.3–0.6 mg intravenously.
   Rationale: This drug increases the heart rate by blocking the effect of parasympathetic nervous activity on the SA node. Atropine is given intravenously to ensure rapid effect.

c Ensure rest and minimize activity. Anticipate and cater for all patient's needs.
   Rationale: This is to reduce the workload of the heart.

d Give oxygen at high concentration via face mask or endotracheal tube if patient is intubated.
   Rationale: This is to ensure that the arterial oxygen level is high enough to maintain tissue perfusion.

e Ensure that emergency resuscitation equipment and drugs are near at hand.
   Rationale: Reduced cardiac output may lead to cardiac arrest or other serious dysrhythmias. (Detect changes in patient's cardiac status).

f Measure and record ECG by cardiac monitor.
   Rationale: This is to detect dysrhythmias and permit prompt treatment.

g Measure and record blood pressure, pulse rate and volume, respiratory rate and pattern, and temperature. This should be done as frequently as the patient's condition indicates.
   Rationale: Blood pressure, pulse rate and volume improve as cardiac output returns to normal. Respirations return to normal as acidosis is corrected. Temperature may rise, this

may be a sign of the inflammatory response from damaged tissue in the myocardium.

Careful assessment and examination of the patient with reduced cardiac output is necessary to prevent potential circulatory fluid overload, which would in turn cause left ventricular heart failure and exacerbate shock.

Nursing assessment would include not only observations of the patient's circulatory function, i.e., blood pressure and pulse, but also their respiratory function. The presence of symptoms of pulmonary oedema must be reported and treated promptly to prevent further compromise to cardiac function. Dyspnoea, hypoxia and haemoptysis may be the presenting symptoms of pulmonary oedema, as are sweating, pallor and anxiety. Crepitations and rhonchi may be heard all over the lung fields.

NURSING INTERVENTIONS FOR THE PATIENT WITH CIRCULATORY OVERLOAD

The objective would be to prevent fluid overload occurring in the first place. Promotion of a normal circulating volume and support of myocardial function are priorities.

1 Measure and record fluid input/output. Report findings if abnormal.

   Monitor fluid balance to ensure correct assessment of fluid requirements. Monitor kidney function for renal output diminishes with shock, aldosterone and the antidiuretic hormone are also released during shock and cause retention of sodium (Na^+) ions and water (H_2O).

2 Observe for signs of oedema in dependent sites of the body, (e.g. sacrum, ankles etc) and raised jugular venous pressure. Careful observation will ensure prompt treatment of over-hydration and relief of symptoms. If breathing spontaneously, the patient will need to sit upright to help breathing.

3 Measure and record central venous pressure, if possible. Central venous pressure monitoring reflects the pressure within the right atrium, and is a good guide to assessment of fluid balance. See Chapter 4. The central venous pressure is raised in pulmonary oedema and fluid overload and de-

creased in hypovolaemia. A normal range of parameters would be +/−2.

4 Coping with the patient and their relatives anxiety. This topic will be fully dealt with in Chapter 9, but suffice it to say at this point that reduction of anxiety will reduce heart work load, make the patient feel better and promote confidence in the staff and help gain patient co-operation.

Give a full explanation to the patient, as his/her condition warrants, and to the relatives. Allow the patient and relatives time to voice their fears, and give opportunity for them to see medical and senior nursing staff. Always inform the patient prior to carrying out procedures and give reassurance and support even when it may not appear to be needed.

SINUS TACHYCARDIA

The impulse originates in the SA node and is conducted normally. The rate is greater than 100 beats per minute and may be as high as 150 beats per minute. The rhythm is regular and the P waves are normal in shape. The P-R interval and QRS complexes are also normal.

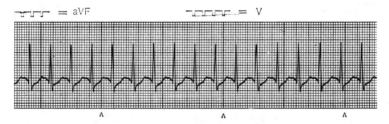

Figure 2.3 *Sinus tachycardia.*

Sinus tachycardia may be present as a result of anxiety or following exercise. Other common causes are pyrexia and pain. It may however herald the onset of haemorrhage, hypoxia, congestive cardiac failure, left ventricular failure or overdosage of certain drugs (these include atrophine, adrenaline, aminophyline or isoprenaline).

Sinus tachycardia, per se, should not be treated. It is a protective, coping mechanism which is part of the fight/flight response to stress. However, sustained heart rates of over 140 beats per minute reduce the cardiac output by decreasing the ventricular filling time, thus reducing stroke volume and shortening diastole. Reduced cardiac output associated with poor tissue perfusion and increased demand on the heart also causes reduced myocardial blood flow, giving rise to ischaemia and pain. Treatment of the cause is important, therefore patient assessment should be directed towards trying to determine why the patient has a tachycardia. It cannot be emphasized enough how important it is to give appropriate support and reassurance to alleviate anxiety, as anxiety is a potent cause of sinus tachycardia.

Potential Problems

Pain

Patient Goal—The patient will experience relief of pain.

Nursing Interventions

1 Administer prescribed drug therapy, observe and report response.
   Rationale: Maintenance of analgesia reduces awareness of pain. It has a sedative calming effect, which helps to reduce heart workload and rate of heart beat.
2 Give psychological support
   Rationale: This will reduce anxiety and stress which in turn will reduce the workload of the heart.
3 Change patients position in bed as appropriate, ensuring support for limbs.
   Rationale: Comfortable positioning in bed promotes rest, reduces heart workload and anxiety.

Hypoxia

Patient Goal—To maintain arterial blood gases within normal limits.

Nursing Interventions

1 Give oxygen at high concentration via face mask, endotracheal tube etc., as prescribed by physician.
  Rationale: This ensures that the arterial oxygen level is high enough to maintain tissue perfusion.
2 If the patient is dyspnoeic, sit them upright and support with pillows. Monitor respirations and report significant changes to the medical staff.
  Rationale: Respiratory capacity is optimized in this position.

Other potential causes of sinus tachycardia should be identified and treated, e.g. haemorrhage should be controlled and fluid replacement given. Pulmonary oedema and heart failure may also be implicated as a cause of sinus tachycardia. Nursing intervention would be similar to treatment of circulatory overload.

SINUS ARRYTHMIA

The impulse originates in the SA node. The rate can be between 60–100 beats per minute, and usually irregular. It can be seen that with respiration, the heart rate accelerates and then slows down in rhythm. Inspiration increases the heart rate, expiration slows it. It is common in young people, and is caused by reflex actions connected to breathing, and in particular, parasympathetic activity from the vagus nerve. The P waves, P-R interval, and QRS complexes are normal in shape. The patient will probably be unaware of this rhythm, and it requires no treatment.

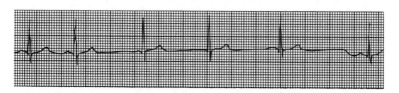

Figure 2.4 *(a) Sinus arrythmia.*

SINUS ARREST — THE MISSED OR DROPPED BEAT!

Sinus arrest is a breakdown in the timing mechanism of the pacemaker in which the SA node periodically 'forgets' to discharge an impulse. As the atria and ventricules do not receive any current they cannot contract. The sensation of the missed beat is noticeable to the patient.

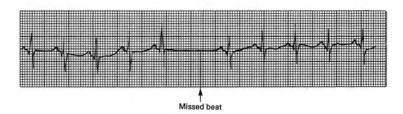

Missed beat

Figure 2.4 *(b) Sinus arrest.*

When observing sinus arrest it should be noted that the return of a normal sinus rhythm is not always at the point where the missed beat should be, this gives the appearance of an irregular rhythm.

The P waves, P-R interval and QRS are of normal shape, although absent at the missed beat. In some cases other cells within the myocardium begin to deputize for the SA node, by originating their own impulse to fill in the gap. This impulse is not of the usual shape, and is called an ectopic or escape beat. The ectopic may not appear in the ECG at the position where the missed beat should be. Ectopic beats may not only originate in the atria, but can start at any area of myocardium, the resulting shape of this ectopic beat will be unusual, normally referred to as bizarre.

If the rate is normal and the cardiac output is maintained, the patient will be unaffected apart from the awareness of the dropped beat. If a bradycardia is present however, the cardiac output may be jeopardized giving rise to symptoms of shock. Sinus arrest may be associated with a number of causes, including ischaemic heart disease, digoxin toxicity, and increased parasympathetic activity.

The Vagus nerve serves a large part of the thorax and abdomen and stimulation of this nerve will stimulate a parasympathetic response. Parasympathetic nerve activity tends to cause slowing of the heart by blocking the action of the SA node. As will be seen later, deliberate stimulation of the parasympathetic nerves can be used to slow down an accelerated heart rate.

Treatment of sinus arrest is related to cause, e.g. if it is due to digoxin toxicity, the drug would be stopped until symptoms subside. Active treatment of this rhythm includes Atropine 0.3–0.6 mg intravenously and, if necessary, insertion of a transvenous pacemaker.

Nursing interventions would include: observation and monitoring of myocardial function. Minimizing patient activity and promoting rest, administering drug therapy and recording response, support and reassurance to the patient and relatives.

WANDERING PACEMAKER

The impulses constantly change sites of origin within the atria, and the AV node may also initiate impulses in this rhythm. This constant change of pacemaker site gives an irregular pattern to the rhythm. The rate is normal, and the P waves vary in shape depending on where the impulse originates. The P-R interval will also change, ranging from 0.2 seconds at the SA node to 0.12 seconds at the AV node. Conduction down the ventricular bundles is normal, and therefore the QRS complexes are normal. This rhythm may be caused by increased parasympathetic activity, ischaemic heart disease or digoxin therapy.

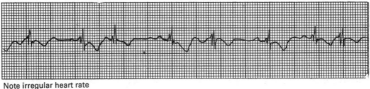

Note irregular heart rate

Figure 2.4   *(c) Wandering pacemaker.*

The patient may have no symptoms, and treatment will only be necessary if the heart rate is very low. Atropine is the drug of choice for this condition. Nursing interventions are as for sinus tachycardia and sinus arrest.

PREMATURE ATRIAL CONTRACTIONS, ECTOPICS

Atrial ectopics originate in an excitable area of atrial tissue which discharges impulses irregularly. The presence of ectopic beats may be a sign of atrial irritability. As the impulse originates outside the SA node, the P wave is abnormally shaped, and the P-R interval may be short or prolonged, depending on where the impulse is initiated. The impulse is conducted down the usual pathways into the ventricles, therefore the QRS complexes will be normal.

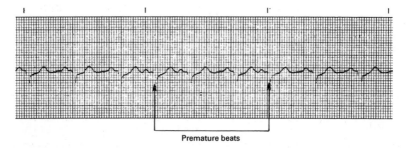

Premature beats

Figure 2.5 *Premature atrial contractions.*

Following an ectopic beat, the SA node which will have depolarized with the rest of the atrial tissue, will need time to recover before discharging the next beat. Recovery by the SA node causes a pause on the ECG trace. This is called the incomplete compensatory pause, and occurs prior to the next sinus beat.

The atrial ectopic beat has no particular significance although it may herald other serious dysrhythmias like atrial fibrillation. Atrial ectopics occurring at a frequency greater than 8/10 per minute must be reported to medical staff. The patient will be unaware of the presence of this dysrhythmia.

Treatment of choice would be digoxin, unless the dysrhythmia was paradoxically caused by this drug, which is possible. Nursing intervention revolves around observation and monitoring of cardiac rhythm and output. See care plan for sinus tachycardia.

ATRIAL FLUTTER

Atrial flutter results from increased atrial ectopic activity and is a sign of atrial irritability. The cells within the atrial myocardium discharge impulses at a very fast rate, 250–350 beats per minute. The AV node cannot relay all the impulses as the rate is too fast. It therefore selects which impulses it wants to conduct, and ignores those it doesn't. This is a form of block. The conduction of impulses to the ventricles is via the normal pathways, and is usually in a regular pattern, e.g. the AV node conducts every second, third, or fourth impulse it receives.

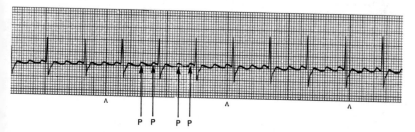

Figure 2.6   *Atrial flutter.*

Examples of atrial versus ventricular rate

It is possible that the atrial rate may be 300, yet the ventricular rate is 150, the AV conduction block is then referred to as 2:1. If it's 3:1 block, the ventricular rate would be 100, and if 4:1 the ventricular rate would be 75 given an atrial rate of 300.

The ventricular rate ranges from 60–160 beats per minute and is usually regular, but as with everything there are exceptions! The blocking action of the AV node can change occasionally giving a irregular rate.

The P waves will be abnormally shaped, and due to the fast atrial rate, will be seen as a saw tooth pattern, characteristic of atrial flutter. This pattern makes identification of single P waves impossible. The saw tooth pattern is made up of flutter waves (F waves) which are the combined electrical activity of the atria. The P-R interval is absent, but the QRS complexes are normal.

If the ventricular rate is rapid, e.g. greater than 140 beats per minute, there will be a reduction in cardiac output giving symptoms of shock. See page 67. The patient may complain of palpitations, angina or dyspnoea due to heart failure or ischaemia. A number of disease processes predispose to atrial flutter, including ischaemic heart disease, congestive cardiac failure, rheumatic heart disease and thyrotoxicosis.

Where facilities are available the treatment of choice is low voltage DC synchronized defibrillation performed under general anaesthetic. This procedure floods the heart muscle with electrical current and eradicates the ectopic activity converting the heart rate to a normal rhythm. Drug therapy may also be used. Verapamil, an agent which specifically inhibits the passage of calcium ions across transmembranes into the myocardial cells, or digoxin are the drugs of choice.

Nursing intervention: Discussion of the nursing interventions required are located at the end of the section on atrial fibrillation.

ATRIAL FIBRILLATION

This rhythm resembles that of atrial flutter, although the atrial rate is much faster, e.g. greater than 360 beats per minute, and the saw tooth appearance is absent. This atrial ectopic activity is uncoordinated and bombards the AV node which cannot cope with this vast number of impulses. The AV node therefore blocks most of them and conducts only some of them in a spasmodic fashion. The ventricular rate is therefore irregular. This frenetic atrial activity is said to resemble a bag of worms. The ineffective atrial contraction fails to fully fill the ventricles with blood prior to their contraction. This will reduce stroke volume by anything up to 20%, and will lead to diminished cardiac output.

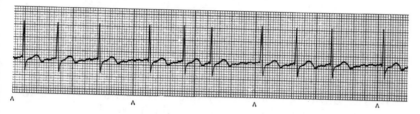

Figure 2.7   *Atrial fibrillation.*

Some of the ventricular contractions produce such a low volume output that the corresponding beat is absent at the radial pulse. It is important to know what the actual effective pulse rate is. To do this, the apex beat, heard through a stethoscope, and the radial pulse, are counted simultaneously. The results gives the:

pulse deficit – the difference in rate between these pulses

In atrial fibrillation it is not usually possible to pick out distinct P waves on the ECG trace and the P-R interval is therefore absent. The QRS complexes are normal in shape but are irregular.

The patient may be aware of the irregular heart rate and complain of palpitations. If the ventricular rate remains rapid, signs of left ventricular failure may be present. The elderly patient may well be symptomless if the ventricular rate is within normal limits and the rhythm is of long standing duration. Drug therapy may be used initially, Digoxin being the drug of choice. Digoxin causes increased blocking of impulses at the AV node, stabilizing the ventricular rate. In some cases verapamil may be used. If atrial fibrillation is persistent, or signs of heart failure or angina develop, the rhythm should be converted rapidly by synchronized D.C. low voltage defibrillation under general anaesthetic. Ineffective contraction of the atria may give rise to stagnation of blood in the atria, leading to the formation of emboli which may be released into the general circulation. This is a serious complication of this rhythm.

CARDIOVERSION, SYNCHRONIZED D.C. DEFIBRILLATION

Cardioversion is a planned procedure, by which a low voltage D.C. current is passed through the chest wall, aimed at causing depolarization of all myocardial tissue. This suppresses atrial ectopic activity and permits the SA node to resume control as the pacemaker of the heart. This technique is used to convert supraventricular tachyarrhythmias where the fast heart rate compromises cardiac output.

Synchronous defibrillation prevents delivery of the current during the recovery period following the QRS complex, the T wave. The T wave is electrically vulnerable and ventricular fibrillation may result if the R wave of the shock is delivered at the T wave of the QRS complex (R on T phenomenon).

This technique is performed under general anaesthesia. The voltage required to convert the rhythm is often much less than that used for emergency defibrillation. The general principles applied to this procedure are the same as those used in emergency defibrillation, except that the patient is anaesthetized. See page 47 for emergency defibrillation.

Before the charge is built up and released the synchronization button is switched on. The current is delivered when the defibrillator senses the patient's own R wave. In this way the T wave portion of the ventricular complex is missed. Complications of this technique include cardiac arrest and skin burns.

Nursing Interventions

Preparation of the patient for cardioversion is an important nursing role. As has been stated it is a planned procedure, and the nurse must consider equally the patient's physiological and psychological needs.

The technique should be carefully explained to the patient, but the patient may have a little time, before cardioversion, to think about its consequences. (The technique involves electrocution, an unpleasant prospect for the patient to face). Anxiety and fear will exacerbate the patient's underlying condition, giving rise to tachycardia and hypertension. It should be remembered that anxiety provokes the stress response, i.e. release of adrenaline. The patient will be suffering a considerable amount of stress and every effort must be made to reassure and support the patient to minimize stress effects on the heart.

The procedure is carried out under general anaesthesia, and the patient must be thoroughly prepared in accordance with hospital protocols. Food and drink should be withheld for at least four hours prior to the procedure, although in a situation where the patient is experiencing reduced cardiac output, this may not be possible. The patient, or relatives, will be required to sign a consent form, before the procedure is performed.

Once the patient is anaesthetized, the defibrillator electrodes are attached to the patient's chest. Care must be taken to ensure that electrode gel, if used, is not smeared across the chest, as this forms a bridge between the two defibrillator paddles and causes a short circuit. If such a situation occurs, a flash of light may be seen and the patient may suffer chest burns due to the electric charge crossing the surface of the chest before running to earth. This situation is particularly dangerous for staff standing nearby who may be electrocuted. Ensure a satisfactory ECG trace is present so that the defibrillator can distinguish where to discharge correctly. Before delivery of the charge, the operator must ensure that all staff are not in contact with the bed.

The preferred and standard positions of the paddles are:

One paddle, in the area of the 2nd intercostal space, right side of the chest.

One paddle, 5th intercostal space, midclavicular line, left side of the chest.

Once the heart rhythm is converted to a more acceptable one, the electrode gel or pads are removed and the patient is placed in the coma position, extubated and allowed to recover from the anaesthetic. The heart rhythm is monitored continuously. Frequent recordings of vital signs and level of consciousness are made until the patient recovers. The nurse must document the number of times defibrillation was performed and the voltages used.

SUPRAVENTRICULAR TACHYCARDIA

This term is a general label for a fast ventricular rhythm originating from somewhere within the myocardium above the ventricles. The rate is 160–200 beats per minute. The rhythm is regular, P waves cannot be seen and P-R interval is absent. The QRS complexes are normal.

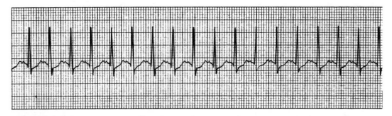

Figure 2.8 *Supraventricular tachycardia.*

The patient may exhibit signs of heart failure and shock. Angina and palpitations may also be present. The predisposing factors to supraventricular tachycardia are ischaemic heart disease, sympathetic nervous activity or drugs.

Treatment includes prevention and correction of shock and the administration of oxygen to counteract hypoxia. Stimulation of the parasympathetic nerve tissue can reduce heart rate, and this may be effected by massage of the carotid sinus body in the neck or supra orbital pressure which may then convert the heart rate to a normal rhythm. If this procedure is used, the patient must be closely monitored as bradycardia or even cardiac standstill are possible complications! Synchronized low voltage D.C. defibrillation may also be used to convert this rhythm. An alternative approach involves drug therapy in the form of beta blockers, e.g. Practolol 10 mg intravenously (N.B. given slowly).

PAROXYSMAL ATRIAL TACHYCARDIA

This rhythm originates in an ectopic focus within the atria. The rate is rapid 150–250 beats per minute. The ectopic rate overcomes the SA node, and the ectopic focus becomes the pacemaker. The impulses are conducted down the usual pathway and the ventricles respond to each impulse. This rhythm occurs without warning, and may stop as suddenly, sometimes without treatment.

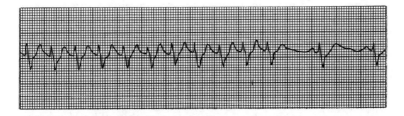

Figure 2.9   *Paroxysmal atrial tachycardia.*

The P waves are abnormal in shape and, because of the fast rate, are buried in the previous T wave. The P-R interval cannot be measured due to the obscured P waves, and the QRS complexes will be normal.

The patient is usually aware of the onset of the rhythm and feels a fluttering sensation in the chest. Syncope, lightheadedness and angina might also be present. Treatment is the same as for supraventricular tachycardia. Once the rhythm has been suppressed prophylactic antiarrythmic drugs are usually prescribed.

JUNCTIONAL RHYTHMS

The AV node does not initiate impulses itself, but the surrounding tissue does. Nodal rhythms refer to impulses originating in this junctional tissue. The junctional tissue only initiates impulses if the atrial pacemaker does not discharge impulses at a rate greater than 60 beats per minute. The impulse originating in the junctional tissue travels into the atria by the normal pathways but backwards! This is called retrograde conduction. Passage of the impulse down the ventricular tissue is in the normal manner.

There are three main areas around the AV node which usually are responsible for initiating impulses.

1 High Nodal: The atria have time to depolarize before the impulse reaches the ventricles, but because the impulse travels backwards, the P wave is inverted.

2 Mid Nodal: The atria and ventricles depolarize together. The muscle mass is greatest in the ventricles and so the P wave is swamped by the ventricular contraction.

3 Low Nodal: The impulse reaches the ventricles before the atria, the P wave is seen after the QRS complex but before the T wave. The P wave will be inverted as in number 1. (See Figure 2.10).

The rate of junctional rhythm is 40 to 65 beats per minute, although junctional tachycardia is possible. The rhythm is regular, P waves may be absent or inverted, and they may appear before or after the QRS complex. P-R interval is variable or absent, and the QRS complex is usually normal.

Ischaemic heart disease, increased sympathetic and para-sympathetic nerve activity, congestive cardiac failure, hypoxia and some cardiac drugs may predispose to junctional rhythms.

As with all dysrhythmias, cardiac output may be compromised and require support. Atropine 0.3–0.6 mg, or isoprenaline by infusion are the drugs of choice. Transvenous pacing may be required if the ventricular rate is very fast.

The nursing interventions for the patient are geared to prompt assessment of the patient's specific needs, prompt reporting and treatment. Rhythms starting in the junctional tissue tend to be unstable, the pacemaker site may 'slip' down into the ventricles, seriously compromising the heart rate, which may fall to 20–40 beats per minute, hence the need for close nursing observation.

Junctional tachycardia, like supraventricular tachycardia, is of two types: constant and paroxysmal. The constant variety has a rate of 70 to 130 beats per minute. This is faster than the AV node's intrinsic rate, but slower than a supraventricular tachycardia which has a rate of 160–200 beats per minute. As a result, junctional tachycardia is now termed accelerated junctional rhythm.

(a)

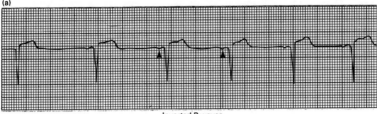

Inverted P waves

(b)   Inverted P waves

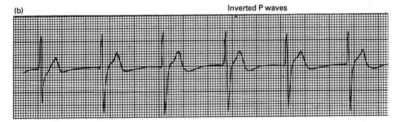

(c)

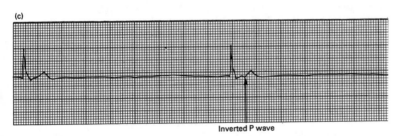

Inverted P wave

Figure 2.10   *(a) High nodal rhythm*
(b) Mid nodal rhythm
(c) Low nodal rhythm.

Paroxysmal junction tachycardia, or paroxysmal accelerated junctional rhythm, is 140–200 beats per minute and is
easily confused with supraventricular tachycardia.

VENTRICULAR ECTOPICS

The impulse originates in the ventricular muscle. Like the
atrial ectopic beat it is an unscheduled beat arriving prema-
turely before the next sinus beat is due, and is followed by a

compensatory pause. The conduction of the impulse is aberrant, unusual and retrograde, and as a result, the QRS wave form is wide and bizarre in shape e.g. greater than 0.12 seconds. The T wave is often in a different direction to the QRS complex.

Ventricular ectopics can be divided into five main types, all of which are potentially dangerous.

1 The isolated single ectopic.
2 Bigemini—The ventricular ectopic alternates with a sinus beat to form a coupled rhythm.
3 R on T—The ventricular ectopic depolorizes on the T wave of a preceding complex. The T wave is electrically unstable and vulnerable to this type of attack, which may provoke the critical condition of ventricular fibrillation.
4 Multifocal ectopics—This shows that ectopic activity is well established and indicates myocardial instability. The ectopic beats arise from different sites within the ventricles, and they therefore differ in shape.
5 Coupled or consecutive ectopics—The ectopics appear together in close proximity. They denote ventricular vulnerability to tachycardia and fibrillation.

In addition to these types of ventricular ectopics, it is also possible for isolated or unifocal ectopics to occur. They should be reported if they occur more than six times per minute as this may herald more serious ventricular dysrhythmias. It has been estimated that 90 per cent of patients develop ventricular ectopics after acute myocardial infarction. Digoxin and hypokalaemia may also precipitate ventricular ectopics.

Symptoms range from none to palpitation and collapse. A standard medical intervention consists of administering the drug of choice lignocaine by bolus injection 50–100 mg intravenously, or by infusion at 2–4 mg per minute.

Nursing intervention would include close observation and reporting of dysrhythmia. The presence of physical symptoms will indicate deterioration in cardiac function.

VENTRICULAR TACHYCARDIA

The ectopic impulses are generated within the ventricular myocardium. The rate is between 140–220 beats per minute.

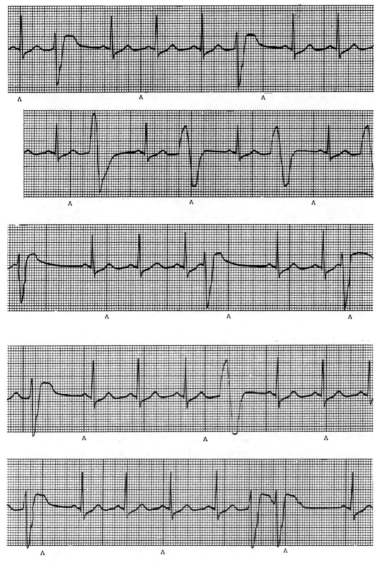

Figure 2.11   (a) Unifocal ventricular ectopics
   (b) Ventricular ectopics: bigemini
   (c) Ventricular ectopics: R on T phenomenon
   (d) Multifocal ventricular ectopics
   (e) Ventricular ectopics: coupled beats.

The rhythm is irregular. P waves are swamped by the QRS complex and are not visible. The QRS complexes are wide and bizarre in shape, greater than 0.12 seconds duration, (See Figure 2.12).

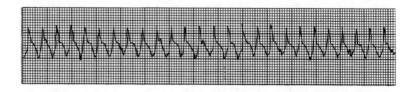

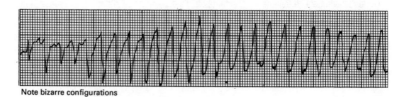

Note bizarre configurations

Figure 2.12 *Ventricular tachycardia.*

Ventricular tachycardia (VT) may occur without warning, but is usually preceded by frequent ventricular ectopics. The rhythm may appear as short 'salvo's' or be sustained. Sustained ventricular tachycardia produces serious cardiovascular effects and it may deteriorate to ventricular fibrillation.

The effects of ventricular tachycardia on the patient are rapid collapse of cardiac output, with associated cardiogenic shock, myocardial and cerebral ischaemia, and possibly sudden death. Signs and symptoms include palpitation, lightheadedness and angina. The patient may experience pronounced anxiety and a feeling of impending doom, not altogether unfounded.

Treatment depends on the patient's level of consciousness. If they are conscious, lignocaine, 50–100 mg is given intravenously (1 mg per kg body weight). If this suppresses the ventricular tachycardia and restores a normal rhythm, a continuous prophylactic infusion of lignocaine, 2–4 mg per minute is indicated.

If the patient is unconscious, emergency D.C. defibrillation is required with a charge of 200 joules. This can be used repeatedly to convert persistent tachycardia. If the rhythm does not convert, cardiac output will virtually be non existent, and external chest compression and ventilation of the lungs with oxygen must be commenced to sustain life. Lignocaine infusion may be used to prevent further episodes of this rhythm.

For nursing care see cardioversion. At this point the nurse should consider the implications of this procedure for the patient. In certain situations the patient experiencing VT may not lose consciousness quickly, they may be aware of the change in their heart rhythm and have feelings of faintness and anxiety. Small doses of sedation i.e. Diazemuls 2–5 mg intravenously will help to lessen their anxiety as will reassurance from the nurse.

It is important to say that patients who have experienced emergency defibrillation and chest compressions will probably remain frightened and apprehensive. They will worry that it may recur, and in some cases the patient may have some memory of the events that have taken place. Frank discussion about the patient's fears will help the nurse to tailor her care to meet the patients special needs.

VENTRICULAR FIBRILLATION

The impulses are generated from many sites within the ventricles. The rate is in excess of 300 beats per minute. Each muscle fibre has no time to recover from the previous depolarization and the result is a general twitching instead of a coordinated contraction of the myocardium. This situation causes collapse of blood pressure and cardiac output. Approximately three minutes later, cerebral hypoxia and metabolic acidosis cause irreparable brain damage.

The rhythm seen on ECG is chaotic and without coordinated ventricular activity. P waves, P-R interval and QRS complexes are absent. Ventricular fibrillation is defined as coarse or fine, depending on the amplitude of the ventricular activity. Coarse fibrillation is easier to convert to a less dangerous rhythm as the electrical activity present is of a sufficient strength to respond well to defibrillation.

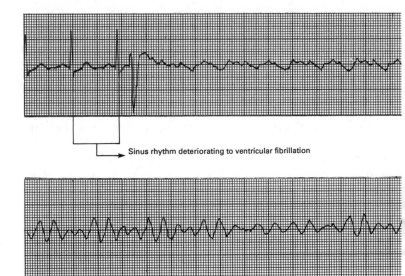

Figure 2.13   *Ventricular fibrillation.*

Management of Ventricular Fibrillation

This is an emergency situation, cardiac output will be non-existent and cerebral hypoxia and poor tissue perfusion will kill the patient within minutes. Full resuscitation with external chest compression and ventilation must commence immediately. Emergency defibrillation at 200 joules must be used to convert the heart rhythm to one which can provide cardiac output. Repeated D.C. shocks can be administered until a rhythm with output is produced. Correction of acidosis can be accomplished by the administration of sodium bicarbonate following arterial blood gas estimation. A high P_{co2} can be treated with intermittent positive pressure ventilation.

The patient will be noted to be in a collapsed state. The nurse should try to find the carotid pulse and observe the patient for signs of breathing which may be absent. The patient is positioned flat and external chest compression commenced. If emergency resuscitation equipment is not immediately at hand, mouth to mouth breathing must begin. The ratio of breaths to cardiac massage is 15 chest compressions to two breaths. ECG monitoring will show the rhythm to be ventricular fibrillation. The treatment required will be D.C. defibrillation at 200 joules, if this does not convert the rhythm, a second shock is delivered at 400 joules, if necessary a 50–100 mg intravenous injection of lignocaine is given followed by a further D.C. shock of 400 joules. If available, bretylium tosylate should be given to promote stabilization of the myocardium, followed by D.C. shock of 400 joules. D. C. defibrillation should be continued until the rhythm is converted to a less dangerous one, or the procedure is ordered to be abandoned by medical staff.

It is important that cardiopulmonary resuscitation should continue between D.C. defibrillations to maintain cardiac output and cerebral blood flow. It is also important that nursing staff should be conversant with the defibrillator and its functions. In an emergency situation the highest charge is used on the defibrillator, on some this may be 360 joules, on others 400. The 400 joule charge is used in this text for example only.

Part of the nurses role is to ensure patient safety, D.C. defibrillation must be carried out safely, or the procedure takes on dangers for staff as well as the patient.

- Ensure that water and other fluids are kept away from the area of the defibrillator, as this may lead to a short circuit and the danger of electrocution.
- Ensure that staff members are not in contact with the patient or bed during defibrillation as they too will receive a shock.
- Ensure that electrode jelly is placed on the defibrillator paddles, this improves contact with the skin and helps to prevent burns. Pre-gelled pads are widely available and are somewhat safer to use.
- Electrode gel can run and if two areas of electrode gel join, then the D.C. current will flow over these sites instead of through the chest. This is called arcing, and causes severe burns. A flash of current may also be seen between the defibrillator paddles.

In summary, direct current defibrillation is a very useful tool but it can be dangerous for both patient and staff if not used correctly.

Defibrillation in emergency situations can be performed by nursing staff who have received appropriate training, the procedure is usually listed under the extended role of the nurse. Training and supervision of nurses undertaking the technique is either by medical or senior nursing staff, who are listed by their hospital as designated trainers.

ASYSTOLE

The ECG will show no signs of electrical activity. After searching for the carotid pulse and quickly assessing the patient for evidence of respiration, the nurse must commence cardiopulmonary resuscitation immediately. The patient should be intubated, as quickly as possible with an endotracheal tube, as this allows improved oxygenation of the lungs and provides a means of suctioning sputum and other detritus which may be blocking the air passages. In the interim, an ordinary oropharyngeal airway should be used to facilitate maintenance of a clear airway during resuscitation.

The first drug to have ready is atropine, 0.3–1.2 mg, to be given intravenously. The second drug of choice is adrenaline, 10 ml of 1:10,000. If this fails to initiate cardiac action, then a further dose may be given.

Sodium bicarbonate, 50 ml of 8.4%, every 20 minutes of the cardiac arrest is sometimes given, although arterial blood gases must be taken to assess whether the patient requires it. Over infusion of sodium bicarbonate can cause metabolic alkalosis a situation nearly as difficult to correct as the metabolic acidosis that occurs in the cardiac arrest situation.

VENTRICULAR STANDSTILL

Total absence of ventricular activity. Atrial activity will be present. The atrial rate will be normal, the ventricular rate will be absent. The absence of ventricular function causes dramatic loss of cardiac output, this is an emergency procedure and is treated as for cardiac arrest.

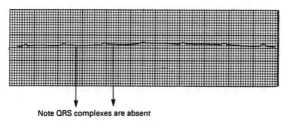

Note QRS complexes are absent

Figure 2.14 *Ventricular standstill.*

ELECTROMECHANICAL DISASSOCIATION

In this situation there is cardiac electrical activity but no cardiac output. Treatment is as for cardiac arrest.

Cardiopulmonary resuscitation can maintain the cardiac output sufficiently to maintain cerebral blood flow for up to an hour or more, the nurse should make every effort to familiarize herself with the techniques involved and to undergo regular practice sessions with a manikin.

COMMON DYSRHYTHMIAS — EXERCISES

1 What are the causes of sinus tachycardia?
2 How would you recognize atrial flutter and what disease processes predispose to this arrhythmia?
3 When would atropine be used and how does it work?
4 Is SVT regular or irregular?
5 What do you understand by the R on T phenomenon?
6 When is synchronized D.C. shock used?
7 What are the five main categories of ventricular ectopics?
8 What do you understand by retrograde conduction and when does it occur?
9 When is verapamil used?
10 When is lignocaine used?

3

Atrioventricular Heart Block

This is a general term for disruption or uncoordinated passage of the electrical current generated by the pacemaker. The pacemaker, as has been mentioned, is not necessarily the SA node but any site within the myocardium that initiates ventricular contraction as a result of discharge of electrical activity.

When discussing atrioventricular blocks, the reader may be more familiar with the terms First, Second and Third Degree Heart Block. It is however, easier to classify heart blocks as SA node blocks, atrioventricular or junctional blocks and intraventricular heart blocks. SA node blocks include heart rhythms discussed in Chapter 2, for example, sinus arrest, which is a disorder of impulse formation. Atrioventricular blocks develop due to tissue damage at the site of the junctional tissue which subsequently disrupting electrical conduction.

FIRST DEGREE ATRIOVENTRICULAR NODE BLOCK

The rhythm is generated within the SA node, but it's conduction through the atrioventricular node is slow. The rate is usually within the normal range, i.e. 70–80 beats per minute, and the P waves are normal in shape and regular. The P-R interval is prolonged, i.e. greater than 0.20 seconds. The conduction of the impulse is normal and the QRS complex is therefore a normal shape. The patient is usually unaffected and unaware of the rhythm—it can only be seen on the ECG trace. The condition may be present in an otherwise healthy person, but it can occur as a sign of ischaemic heart disease, following inferior myocardial infarction, or as a result of digoxin or other antiarrythmic drug therapy. Treatment is usually unnecessary.

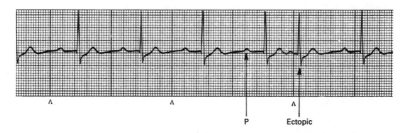

Figure 3.1 *(a) First degree heart block (note prolonged PR interval).*

Problem: First degree heart block.
Goal: Prevent deterioration to more serious dysrhythmia.
Nursing Interventions
1 Observe ECG on frequent basis.
   Rationale: Monitoring P-R interval for progressive lengthening will allow early detection of any deterioration towards a more serious form of block.
2 Record and report changes in rhythm promptly.
   Rationale: Ensures prompt treatment of potentially dangerous dysrhythmia.
3 Discuss administration of anti-arrhythmic drugs with medical staff before giving any such medication.
   Rationale: Ensures atrioventricular conduction is not further depressed.
4 Monitor cardiovascular status (CVS), record and report:
   • blood pressure,
   • pulse volume and rate.
   Rationale: Ensures changes in CVS are observed and recorded promptly.
   • Blood pressure will fall if cardiac output is inhibited
   • Will give warning of slow heart rate (bradycardia),

reduced cardiac output and any potentially lethal ventricular dysrhythmia.

SECOND DEGREE ATRIOVENTRICULAR HEART BLOCK

Type 1: Wenkebach

The impulse is generated in the atrial pacemaker in the usual way but conduction of each impulse progressively becomes more difficult until a beat is dropped, recovery is made, and the cycle then begins again. Commonly it is every 4th or 5th beat that is dropped.

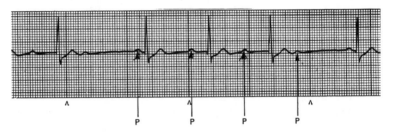

Figure 3.1 *(b) Second degree atrioventricular heart block. Type I: Wenkebach (note progressively lengthening PR interval).*

An analogy can be drawn from the notion of moving furniture: the first piece is easy, but every succeeding piece becomes more difficult to move, until you take a break. Refreshed after the break, you find the next piece of furniture you move is relatively easy.

The P waves are normal in rate and shape. The P-R interval progressively lengthens, until the dropped beat. The QRS complexes are normal in shape, although the ventricular rate may be slow, and absent during the mis-beat. The rhythm is usually transient and often occurs after inferior myocardial infarction. The symptoms may persist for several days or longer. The patient may experience no symptoms, particularly if the ventricular rate is normal. If the rate however, drops below 50 beats per minute, the cardiac output will be reduced or the rhythm may deteriorate to third degree, complete heart block. The symptoms include angina, dyspnoea and light-headedness.

NURSING ROLE

Problem: Second degree heart block, with potential risk of reduced cardiac output.
Goal: The patient will have an adequate circulation until improvement is sustained.
Nursing Interventions: See care plan, first degree heart block, Nos 1–4.

Potential Problem: Compromised cardiac output leading to shock and heart failure.
Goal: Shock or heart failure will not occur.
Nursing Interventions: The aim of nursing care is to support the circulation thereby preventing shock and heart failure.
1 Lie the patient flat with legs elevated.
   Rationale: Ensures good venous return to the heart.
2 Check that resuscitation equipment and drugs are near at hand.
   Rationale: Ensures prompt treatment of life threatening dysrhythmias.
3 Give high concentrations of oxygen by face mask or nasal cannulae.
   Rationale: Maintains arterial oxygen concentration and promotes tissue perfusion.
4 Minimize patient's activity, anticipate and cater for all needs.
   Rationale:
   Reduces demand on the heart.

Problem: Dyspnoea due to heart failure.
Goal: The patient will have a normal respiratory rate.
Nursing Interventions
1 Position upright in bed and support with pillow.
   Rationale: Ensures improved chest expansion by allowing the diaphragm its full range of movement.
2 Give oxygen, as prescribed, by face mask or nasal cannulae.

Rationale: Ensures adequate arterial oxygen concentration and tissue perfusion.
Nasal cannulae are often tolerated better than face masks which tend to cause feelings of suffocation.
3 Observe respiratory rate and pattern, watch particularly for signs of pulmonary oedema: pink frothy sputum (haemoptysis), distention of neck veins and cyanosis.
Rationale: Use of accessory muscles of respiratory may indicate impending respiratory failure.
4 Administer analgesic and diuretic drugs as prescribed.
Rationale: Relieves pain and causes a diuresis which reduces the heart workload.
5 Monitor fluid balance by precise input/output recordings.
Rationale: The anti-diuretic hormone and aldosterone are released during shock and cause oliguria and retention of sodium and water leading to fluid overload. Accurate fluid balance also permits monitoring of kidney function which may be seriously impaired if shock develops.

Problem: Potential risk of third degree (complete) heart block or ventricular standstill.
Goal: Heart rate and cardiac output will be within normal range.
Nursing Interventions
1 Prepare patient for tranvenous pacing.
2 Explain procedure fully to patient and relatives.
Rationale: Alleviates anxiety and reduces fears of the unknown. Ensures confidence in hospital staff and promotes patient cooperation.
3 Ensure consent form is signed.
4 (In ITU or CCU) prepare equipment for insertion of pacing wire. On the ward, ensure X-ray department is notified of impending procedure.
Rationale: Early warning and preparation ensures prompt treatment and improves co-operation with other disciplines, maintaining good lines of communication.

The treatment of second and third degree conduction blocks is primarily by insertion of temporary pacemakers if the patient is symptomatic. Further discussion on the insertion of a pacemaker, and patient management follows at the end of the chapter.

TYPE II, MOBITZ ATRIO-VENTRICULAR CONDUCTION BLOCK

This is a less common dysrhythmia than Type 1, though it is considerably more serious. The impulse is generated in the SA node, its conduction through to the ventricles is blocked below the AV junction tissue, this means that every 2nd, 3rd or 4th sinus beat is not conducted. The terms 2:1, 3:1, or 4:1 block are used depending on the frequency with which a beat is missed.

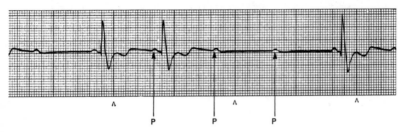

Figure 3.1   (c) Second degree atrioventricular heart block. Type II: Mobitz.

This heart block can occur as a single occasional dropped beat, but if it occurs as a 2:1 block the heart rate is seriously compromised and the cardiac output will be reduced. This rhythm may lead to complete heart block or ventricular standstill. As the block occurs below the junctional tissue, the AV nodal cells cannot take over as a pacemaker. Cardiac output is now dependent on the intrinsic ventricular rate.

The heart rate is usually slow. The P waves are normal, the P-R interval is unchanged and regular until it becomes absent at the dropped beat. The QRS complex is widened as the block appears within the conducting tissue of the ventricles, causing the impulse to be delivered by a roundabout route. The rhythm usually occurs as a result of anterior or anterioseptal infarction. Transvenous pacing may be performed as this rhythm may deteriorate to third degree (complete) heart block. For nursing management see page 53.

THIRD DEGREE HEART BLOCK, COMPLETE ATRIO-VENTRICULAR DISASSOCIATION

In this condition the atria and ventricles depolarize independently of each other consequently the heart can be said to have two pacemakers.

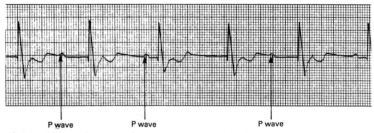

P wave   P wave   P wave

Figure 3.1   *(d)   Complete atrioventricular dissociation.
Third degree heart block.*

An impulse is generated in the SA node, at the usual rate of 70–80 beats per minute, and is conducted through the atrial tissue but does not reach the ventricles. The P waves are therefore regular in shape and rhythm. The ventricular pacemaker is situated below the junctional tissue and its rate is between 20–40 beats per minute. As the impulses arising in the ventricles are conducted through the ventricular tissue in a retrograde way, the QRS complexes are widened and distorted in shape.

The cardiac output is dependent on the ventricular heart rate which will often be insufficient to maintain it at a satisfactory level. Ventricular pacemakers tend to be unreliable and can fail suddenly, allowing ventricular tachycardia, fibrillation or standstill to occur at any time.

The symptoms of light-headedness, angina, syncope and confusion indicate heart failure and reduced cardiac output. The carotid or radial pulse will be slow and regular and will not change with patient activity.

The medical treatment for this condition involves transvenous pacing, meanwhile the patient should be cared for as described in the section on second degree heart block.

BUNDLE BRANCH BLOCK, INTRAVENTRICULAR HEART BLOCK

The conduction pathway below the AV node is called the bundle of His. This conduction tissue divides into two main branches, left and right, each serving one ventricle. The bundle branches are in turn divided into fascicles. The left main bundle branch, divides to form the anterior and posterior fascicles.

Damage to any of the fascicles can be caused by acute myocardial infarction or by chronic scarring and fibrosis. Bundle branch block (BBB) prevents conduction of an impulse to an area of tissue by the usual route, consequently it has to follow an alternative roundabout route which takes longer. The QRS waveform will be widened, e.g. >0.12 seconds, and its shape will be distorted.

The waveform associated with BBB is a characteristic M shape and can only be seen properly on the twelve lead ECG. It is indicative of myocardial damage in many cases.

Blocking of the bundle branches is not confined to the main bundles, but the anterior and posterior fascicles may also be involved, either singly or in combination.

Some of the terms associated with BBB are listed as follows:

RBBB refers to blocking of the right bundle branch.

LBBB refers to blocking of the left bundle branch.

Left Anterior Hemiblock refers to block of the anterior fascicle.

Left Posterior Hemiblock refers to block of the posterior fascicle.

Bifascicular block refers to block of the right bundle branch and one of the fascicles.

Trifascicular block refers to block of all branches.

RBBB

In this condition, impulse conduction down the right bundle branch is blocked, the septum depolarizes from the left and the electric current passes finally into the right ventricle, but not through the usual pathway. The ventricle is therefore slow to react due to the prolonged passage of the impulse. The left ventricle therefore receives its own current first and depolarizes before the right. The M shaped pattern produced on the ECG, best seen in lead V1.

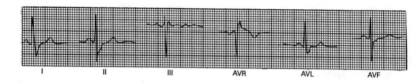

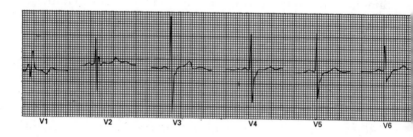

Figure 3.2 *Diagram of right bundle branch block (note notching of R wave in AVR and V₁).*

Right bundle branch block may occur in otherwise healthy people and is not significant if the QRS complex is of normal length, e.g. 0.12 seconds.

LBBB

The impulse is not conducted normally through the left bundle branches. The right ventricle depolarizes first and the left ventricle follows shortly afterwards. The current passes by a roundabout method causing distortion and widening of the QRS waveform.

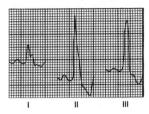

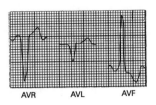

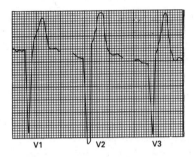

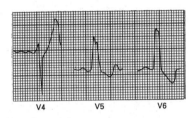

Figure 3.3   *Diagram of left bundle branch block (note notching of R wave in I, II, V₄, V₅, V₆.*

LBBB can best be seen in lead V6, notching of the waveform also can be seen in other leads, especially V5 and V4.

LBBB can disguise the presence of myocardial infarction on the ECG and makes interpretation difficult. It is always significant and indicates an underlying condition such as pulmonary hypertension, ischaemic heart disease or acute pulmonary embolism.

Bundle branch block does not usually cause symptoms although cardiac failure may be present due to slow depolarization of the ventricles reducing cardiac output.

Wolff Parkinson White Syndrome

This is termed a pre-excitation syndrome. An anomalous, or unusual pathway, exists between atria and ventricles and is separate from the AV nodal tissue. This pathway permits an impulse to reach the ventricles, without being relayed through the AV tissue, causing early depolarization. This predisposes the patient to paroxysmal supraventricular tachycardia.

The rate is regular at approximately 100 beats per minute, and the impulses originate in the SA node. The P waves are normal. The P-R interval is short, <0.06 seconds. The QRS is abnormally wide with slurred and notched R waves (Delta waves).

Treatment for the condition is symptomatic and is the same as for supraventricular tachycardia. It is caused by cardiomyopathy or ischaemic heart disease although underlying heart disease may not be apparent.

Stokes Adams Attacks

This term describes intermittent attacks of syncope caused by transient ventricular standstill. It is common in patients who lose ventricular activity due to heart block, e.g. second or third degree.

The attacks are unheralded by dizziness or light-headedness and they may last for up to 30 seconds. The patient is usually shocked and pulseless. The heart beat returns suddenly and the patient regains consciousness. The patient may appear flushed due to capillary dilation from hypoxia. An attack may deteriorate to ventricular tachycardia, fibrillation or cardiac arrest. The attack can occur singly or in succession. Permanent transvenous pacing must be considered.

MYOCARDIAL INFARCTION

Myocardial infarction is caused by ischaemic heart disease and is due to an interruption of the blood supply to myocardial tissue, leading to its death. There are many predisposing factors to myocardial infarction and these include: smoking, obesity, diabetes, hypertension, hyperlipidaemia, stress, poor diet and lack of exercise. There are some indications that personality type may also predispose to myocardial infarction. This condition can be classed with coronary occlusion, thrombosis and atherosclerosis as consequences of ischaemic heart disease.

An anterior infarction causes damage to the anterior, or frontal walls of the ventricles whilst a posterior infarction usually refers to damage in the posterior, or rear part of the ventricles. An inferior-lateral infarction describes damage to the atria and the associated ventricular wall. Anterior myocardial infarctions are significant in that they affect the muscle mass in the ventricle and can reduce the pumping efficiency of the heart with possibly fatal consequences.

Inferior infarctions are significant in that atrial damage predisposes the patient to AV block and can disrupt the conducting pathway of the heart. When discussing myocardial infarction we refer to three distinct types of tissue damage:

1 Necrosis, (tissue death).
2 Injury.
3 Ischaemia.

These can occur simultaneously around the site of infarction. The ECG shows characteristic signs of damage to the myocardium. One of these signs is the presence of deep Q waves, which indicate inert, dead tissue. (See Figure 1.5). Q waves take several days to develop and may therefore not be seen immediately on the ECG. The Q waves will only be present in leads which face the affected area. See page 18.

Tissue near the infarcted area may not be dead but severely damaged. It will conduct impulses but contracts slowly. The effect of this is seen in the S-T segment. The S-T segment will be raised in leads facing the infarction and be depressed in those facing away from it (see page 4). Leads facing away from the site of injury provide a mirror image of what the opposite leads are 'seeing'. This is called a reciprocal change.

The third region within the infarcted area is the ischaemic zone. Here the tissue has an inadequate blood supply and therefore works less efficiently. When infarction has taken place the T wave appears inverted and may form a sharp point due to abnormal repolarization. The T wave is however vulnerable to changes in the electrolyte balance and other variables which makes it unreliable for definitive diagnosis of myocardial infarction. Taken in combination, if Q waves, a raised S-T segment and inverted T waves are present, it is safe to assume myocardial infarction has taken place. Other tests may be necessary to make a firm diagnosis, and one common blood test taken after myocardial infarction is cardiac enzyme assay.

Enzymes are catalysts, they accelerate chemical reactions

within the body. Damage to tissue releases these enzymes into the blood stream. Detection of high levels of cardiac enzymes in isolation is not an infallible method of detecting myocardial infarction as they are also released as a response to trauma to other organs or after cardiac massage.

One common enzyme found following myocardial infarction is SGOT, serum glutamic oxalo-acetic transaminase. After infarction the level rises in the blood until it reaches a peak at 12 to 36 hours. The level in the blood returns to normal in three to five days. It is also found in cerebral, renal and hepatic tissue.

SLDH, serum lactate dehydrogenase is a second common enzyme found in myocardial tissue and red blood cells. This enzyme is released more slowly and reaches a peak at one to two days, it may take up to three weeks to return to normal levels.

The main presenting symptom of myocardial infarction is pain. The patient may experience an unpleasant crushing sensation or describe it as a tight band around the chest. The pain may radiate to both sides of the chest, to the jaw, shoulders and to one or both arms. The pain is not usually brought on by exertion (unlike angina) and usually lasts for more than 30 minutes. It is unrelieved by GTN, (glyceryl trinitrate) or rest distinguishing it from anginal pain.

The complications associated with myocardial infarction are:
1 Cardiogenic shock
2 Respiratory failure
   Heart failure
3 Cardiac dysrhythmias which may be fatal
4 Embolism, pulmonary or cerebral
5 Ventricular aneurysm
6 Rupture of papillary muscles within the heart
7 Post myocardial infarction syndrome, with pericarditis, fever and pleurisy

The ECG shows characteristic changes over a period of time after infarction which may be described as follows.

Acute Infarction, occurring in past few hours shows:
• Deep Q waves
• Raised S-T segment
• Inverted T waves

Recent Infarction, occurring between one and four weeks ago shows:
- Deep Q waves
- Normal S-T segment
- Probably normal T wave, although may still be inverted

Old Infarction, occurring more than four weeks ago:
- Deep Q waves
- Normal S-T segment
- Normal T wave although may still be inverted

The following guidelines set out what to look for when interpreting the ECG for signs of infarction.

Anterior Infarction

Changes, e.g. Q waves, altered S-T segment and inverted T wave, will be seen in all the V leads. Reciprocal changes occur in the standard leads I and aVR.

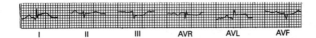

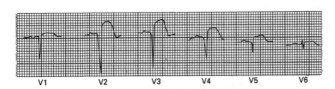

Figure 3.4   *Diagram of anterior myocardial infarction (note elevated ST section in I, V, V_5 with compensatory depression in III).*

Anterior Septal Infarction

Changes appear in leads V1 to V4. Reciprocal changes in standard leads I and aVR.

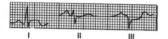

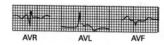

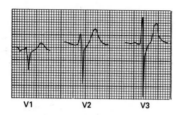

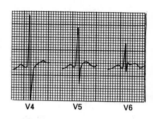

Figure 3.5 *Diagram of an anteroseptal myocardial infarction (note ST elevation in V_1, V_2, V_3 and V_5).*

Anterior Lateral Infarction

Changes occur in leads V4 to V6. Reciprocal changes occur in standard leads I and AVL.

Inferior Infarction

Changes occur in standard leads II, III, and aVF. Reciprocal changes may appear in V leads but usually they are normal.

Inferior Lateral Infarction

Changes occur in standard leads I, aVR, V5 and V6.

Nursing Care of a Patient after Myocardial Infarction

Problem: Pain.
Goal: Patient will experience relief of pain.
Nursing Intervention
Prepare and administer prescribed analgesia, this is usually diamorphine 2.5–5 mg. Intravenous administration of diamorphine is usually a medical intervention unless a specific local unit arrangement has been made under an 'extended role' agreement. An anti-emetic should always be given

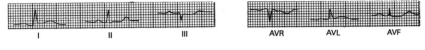

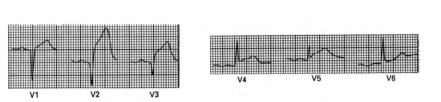

Figure 3.6 *Diagram of an anterolateral myocardial infarction (note ST elevation in AVL, V_5 and V_6).*

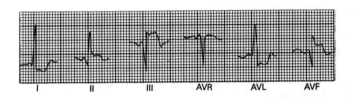

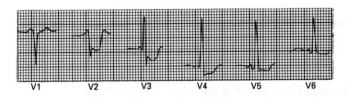

Figure 3.7 *Diagram of an inferior myocardial infarction and reciprocal anterior changes (note ST elevation in II, III and aVF, and depression in AVL, and depression in I, AVL, V_2–V_5).*

prophylactically with intravenous diamorphine, (i.e. 12.5 mg prochlorperazine intramuscularly).

Rationale: Rapid pain relief is achieved by the intravenous route. Narcotic analgesia also promotes patient relaxation and reduces the workload of the heart by reducing anxiety and stress.

Problem: Nausea
Goal: The patient will not feel nauseated.
Nursing Interventions
1 Prepare and administer prescribed anti-emetic. Usually this is prochlorperazine 12.5 mgs.
   Rationale: Nausea is often an associated symptom of myocardial infarction and administration of narcotic analgesic drugs.
2 Remain with patient.
   Rationale: Reassuring for the patient.
3 Provide vomit bowl.
4 Provide mouthwashes frequently.
   Rationale: Removes unpleasant taste of vomit from mouth.

Problem: Patient and relatives' anxiety.
Goal: Patient will state they are less anxious.
Nursing Interventions
1 Give full explanations of patient's condition and treatment.
   Rationale: Gains confidence and compliance of patient and relatives.
2 Give explanations prior to undertaking procedures.
   Rationale: Allows patient time to readjust to situation.
3 Give patient and relatives opportunity to voice fears by active listening.
   Rationale: Reduces fear of the unknown.
4 Give patient and relatives opportunity to talk to medical and nursing staff.
   Rationale: Promotes confidence in hospital staff.
5 Permit relatives to stay close by, advise on visiting, explain the patient's need to rest quietly, restrict visiting only if necessary.
   Rationale: Promotes reassurance and prevents patients and relatives feeling isolated from each other.
6 Encourage involvement of other disciplines, e.g. social workers, or clergy.
   Rationale: Ensures good lines of communication and co-operation between disciplines. Provides adequate support for patient and relatives, reduces their feelings of isolation.

7 Maintain a quiet environment.
  Rationale: Promotes rest and sleep and reduces demand on the heart.

Problem: Shock, due to reduced cardiac output.
Goal: The patient will maintain adequate circulation until improvement occurs in cardiac output as shown by systolic blood pressure greater than 90 mmHg.
Nursing Interventions
1 Position patient flat with legs raised.
  Rationale: Improves cerebral blood flow and helps venous return.
2 The patient may require inotropic drugs by intravenous infusion to support heart function. Administer drugs via infusion pump.
  Rationale: To ensure accurate and continuous administration of the drug. Permit careful titration of dose to patient requirements.
3 Give oxygen at high concentrations by face mask or nasal cannulae.
  Rationale: Maintains arterial oxygen concentration at high level and aids tissue perfusion.
4 Ensure rest and minimize patient activity, anticipate and cater for patient needs.
  Rationale: Reduces heart workload.
5 Ensure emergency resuscitation equipment and drugs are at hand.
  Rationale: Reduced cardiac output may deteriorate to cardiac arrest.
6 Measure and record vital signs:
  • Blood pressure.
  • Pulse, rate and volume.
  • Respiration, rate and pattern, arterial blood gases.
  • Temperature, both core and peripheral.
  • Central venous pressure, and or Swan Ganz monitoring.
  Rationale:
a Blood pressure improves as cardiac output improves, an arterial line permits continuous trend recording of blood pressure to enable accurate doses of inotropic drugs to be administered.

b Pulse rate returns to normal and volume improves with improved cardiac output.
c Respiratory rate and pattern returns to normal as acidosis is corrected by the body. Frequent sampling of arterial blood improves assessment of respiratory and circulatory function.
d Temperature may rise as a sign of the inflammatory response to damaged tissue. A fall in the cardiac output is followed shortly after by peripheral vasoconstriction, the patient may therefore feel cold.
e CVP and/or Swan ganz monitoring/wedge pressures are good indicators of both right and left ventricular functioning.

Problem: Cardiac dysrhythmias.
Goal: Dysrhythmia will not lead to complications for the patient.
Nursing Interventions
1 Continuously monitor cardiac rhythm with oscilloscope.
2 Report changes in rhythm promptly to medical staff.
  Rationale: Permits prompt interventional medical care.

Problem: Potential electrolyte imbalance, e.g. serum potassium.
Goal: Serum electrolytes within normal limits.
Nursing Intervention
Ensure regular monitoring of serum electrolytes.
Rationale: Permit replacement therapy as appropriate.

Problem: Potential circulatory fluid overload. Decreased urine output
Goal: The patient's circulation will not become overloaded. Urine output of 1.5 litres per day.
Nursing Interventions
1 Record precise fluid input/output.
  Rationale: Renal output will diminish with shock. Accurate records will help prevent circulatory fluid overload.
2 Catheterize the patient, if he/she develops retention of urine.
  Rationale: 2 & 3 Permit monitoring of renal function.

Observe for symptoms of pulmonary oedema and notify medical staff, these include:
- Dyspnoea
- Agitation
- Crepitations heard in the chest
- Productive cough, particularly haemoptysis

3 Estimate and record urine output hourly
Rationale: Aldosterone and the anti-diuretic hormone are released during shock, they cause retention of sodium and water. Combined with impaired cardiac function this may cause circulatory fluid overload.

4 Prevent catheter tubing dragging, fix to thigh with tape to secure.
Rationale: Minimizes catheter movement and prevents patient discomfort.

Problem: Potential for ascending urinary infection.
Goal: Patient will not develop urinary tract infection.
Nursing Interventions
1 Maintain closed drainage system.
2 Carry out vulval toilet and catheter care at least six hourly.
Rationale: Reduces risk of ascending infection.
3 Observe for symptoms of ascending urinary infection:
- Rise in temperature,
- Pain, usually lower abdominal,
- Presence of protein and blood in the urine.

Rationale: Permits prompt treatment of infection.

Problem: Sweating
Goal: Patient will not feel uncomfortable due to sweating.
Nursing Interventions
1 Provide cool, dry bed clothes.
2 Permit frequent hands and face washes.
3 Use light bed clothes.
Rationale: Ensures patient comfort.

Problem: Reduced patient activity, inability to attend to own hygiene needs.
Goal: Patient will be satisfied with their personal hygiene
Nursing Interventions
1 Bath in bed daily.

Rationale: Removes sweat and ensures patient comfort.
2 Attend to oral hygiene.
   Rationale: Ensures patient comfort.
3 Gradually increase amount the patient does for themselves in attending to personal hygiene.
   Rationale: Good for patient morale as it helps to restore control over own life.

Problem: Constipation
Goal: The patient will maintain normal bowel function.
Nursing Interventions
1 Ensure fluid intake of minimum two litres a day.
   Rationale: Keeps stools soft.
2 Give aperients and suppositories as required for patient comfort.
   Rationale: Keeps rectum empty.

Potential Problem: Anorexia due to feelings of nausea.
Goal: Daily carbohydrate intake of 2,000 calories.
Nursing Interventions
1 Ensure anti-emetic medication is given.
   Rationale: Counteracts nausea due to narcotic analgesia.
2 Provide suitable light meals and drinks to taste.
   Rationale: Encourages adequate nutrition.
3 Arrange for dietician to see patient and relatives to discuss potential revision of diet and future care.
   Rationale: Prepares the patient for future care, and involves patient in decisions made about his own body.
4 Encourage reduced intake of added salt and fat in the diet.
   Rationale: Helps to reduce the number of predisposing factors the patient has to ischaemic heart disease.
5 Give reducing diet if appropriate.

Potential Problem: Patient smokes
Goal: Patient will give up habit.
Nursing Interventions
1 Give advice and support.
2 Encourage deep breathing and expectoration.
   Rationale: Allows adequate ventilation and perfusion of tissues.

3 Encourage abstinence.
   Rationale: Nicotine causes constriction of blood vessels.

Problem: Decreased mobility due to myocardial infarction.
Goal: Patient will attain at least their previous level of mobility.
Nursing Interventions
1 Encourage gentle, progressive exercise and mobility as patient's condition improves.
   Rationale: Permits the patient to progressively return to normal mobility without straining the heart.
2 Encourage leg exercises, and deep breathing in association with the physiotherapist.
   Rationale: Leg exercises help to prevent venous stasis and potential risk of deep vein thrombosis. Deep breathing exercises promote good lung expansion and maintain arterial oxygenation.

Problem: Patient and relatives anxious about convalescence and rehabilitation at home.
Goal: Family and patient will state they feel able to successfully cope with rehabilitation after discharge.
Nursing Interventions
1 The nurse should be prepared to answer, advise or redirect to appropriate staff, questions the patient may have including exercise tolerance, sex, ability of the patient to return to work and to drive.
   Rationale: Refer to medical or senior nursing staff if unsure or unable to answer patient's questions. Appropriate reassurance and advice alleviates anxiety and fears about going home.
2 Advise on outside agencies the patient or relatives may wish to contact for support and further information.

ANGINA PECTORIS

This is a generalized myocardial ischaemia characterized by poor coronary perfusion and pain. The predisposing factors are the same as for myocardial infarction. Angina is however usually transient pain, associated with exercise, whereas infarction produces prolonged constant pain.

The effects of angina on the ECG are S-T segment depression, or horizontal displacement of 5 mm occurring in all leads. This indicates prolonged conduction of the electrical current, the repolarization is also slower. Between attacks the ECG is usually normal. The attack may last between one and ten minutes, and is brought on by stress or exercise.

The pain is associated with myocardial hypoxia and in addition to ischaemic heart disease; hyperthyroidism and mitral or aortic stenosis are other possible causes. Symptoms are retrosternal pain radiating to particularly the left arm and the angle of the jaw. The pain may be strangling in sensation, or burning.

Treatment includes GTN, by tablet sublingually, or by skin patch. The patient should be encouraged to rest until the attack is over. Improved diet, weight loss and abstinence from smoking will help to prevent re-occurrence of angina.

Transvenous Pacing

If the heart does not generate impulses, or fails to conduct them, stimulation of ventricular contraction can be achieved by electrical impulses from an external battery powered pacemaker.

The pacemaker discharges repetitive electrical currents into a catheter electrode. The catheter is inserted through the subclavian vein into the right ventricle. Temporary pacemakers are installed when heart block is present or during the acute phase of myocardial infarction, and they can be subsequently removed. Long term pacing is instituted for permanent irreversible myocardial damage.

Temporary Pacing

The catheter is passed into the right ventricle where it lodges against the endocardium.

The pacing system consists of two components:

1 The pulse generator which is the source of the impulse. The rate and intensity of the impulses can be regulated by control mechanisms on the pulse generator.

2 An insulated wire catheter carries the impulses from the source to the right ventricle.

The pulse generator can be set in two modes, fixed rate and demand.

Fixed Rate

The pacemaker discharges an impulse at a fixed rate, for example, 60 per minute. The ECG will show regular deflections which are called pacing spikes, these spikes stimulate myocardial depolarization. (See Figure 3.8).

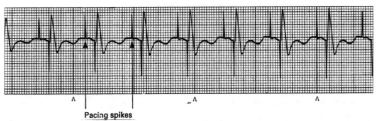

Pacing spikes

Figure 3.8   *An ECG trace showing pacemaker spikes.*

The QRS complex will be wide in shape as the impulse is conducted by an unconventional route.

Disadvantages

At a fixed rate the pacemaker ignores existing electrical activity within the heart and continues to discharge impulses regularly regardless of need. When natural and paced rhythms occur together there is a potential for ventricular dysrhythmia. This is particularly so if the paced beat occurs on the T wave of the previous complex, a period of instability and vulnerability in the myocardium. Ventricular tachycardia or fibrillation can occur. This is a similar situation to R on T ectopics. The potential for ventricular fibrillation is increased in the presence of myocardial ischaemia. It is for this reason demand pacing is preferred for treatment of acute myocardial infarction.

Demand Pacing

This pacemaker does not fire indiscriminately, but only on demand, allowing the natural heart rate to take over where it can. By this means it supports and supplements the natural intrinsic heart rate. The demand pacemaker only discharges an impulse if a QRS complex does not occur within a preset time limit. The pacemaker recognizes natural heart beat by means of an electrode in the pacing wire. When a natural heart beat occurs it is relayed to a sensing device in the pacemaker which inhibits discharge of a pacing impulse.

The pacemaker catheter is inserted under direct X-ray vision, by image intensifier, and with continuous full ECG monitoring. This is usually performed in the X-ray laboratory or department. In emergency situations the pacemaker can be inserted in the CCU with the use of a portable X-ray image intensifier.

Following placement of the catheter the free end is attached to the pacing box. When a pacemaker is inserted it is important the paced heart rate should not be too fast as this increases myocardial oxygen consumption and may cause anginal pain. Too fast a rate reduces ventricular filling time, stroke volume and cardiac output. Paced heart beats encourage efficient heart pumping and suppress dysrhythmias.

Having inserted the pacemaker it is necessary to set it to the correct current i.e. the level of stimulation needed to cause a contraction. If the impulse is not strong enough, contraction does not occur but conversely too strong a stimulus may cause myocardial damage. The heart works on an all or nothing principle, therefore there will be either full ventricular contraction or none at all.

Following insertion the current, is slowly increased until a QRS appears on ECG, this is the threshold. The usual current is approximately 2mA. If the threshold is six to eight, the impulse is very powerful and should stimulate a contraction, if it does not, this usually means the catheter is ruptured or incorrectly positioned. The threshold changes due to movement and other factors, it is therefore important to set the pacemaker with a safety margin to allow for such factors.

Nursing Role

Once set, the nurse must not adjust the pacemaker but should observe the patient for signs of pacemaker failure, initiate immediate treatment for shock, and notify medical staff of the emergency situation.

Problem: Shock associated with loss of pacemaker function.
Goal: The patient will maintain cardiac output until pacing is restored.
Nursing Interventions: As for the nursing care plan for myocardial infarction.
1 Monitor ECG continuously, visualize pacing spike.
  Rationale: Loss of pacing spike artefact means possible catheter fracture.
2 Treat shock.

Potential Problem: Potential haematoma formation or arterial puncture caused by insertion of pacing wire.
Goal: Patient will not become shocked as a result of arterial puncture.
Nursing Interventions
1 Observe blood pressure and pulse for signs of shock.
2 Report findings to medical staff.
3 Implement emergency resuscitation techniques as necessary.
  Rationale: Ensures prompt treatment.

Potential Problem: Pneumo/haemothorax caused by insertion of pacing wire.
Goal: Embarrassment to respiratory function will not occur.
Nursing Intervention
1 Observe respiratory rate, colour and ensure equal chest expansion.
2 Prepare for insertion of chest drain.
  Rationale: Blood in the pleural cavity (haemothorax) may cause compression of the cardiac venous inflow, resulting in dyspnoea and reduced cardiac output.

3 Give oxygen by face mask or nasal cannulae.
   Rationale: Maintains arterial oxygen concentration and ensures tissue perfusion.

Potential Problem: Risk of infection.
Goal: Infection will not occur.
Nursing Interventions
1 Use aseptic technique when dressing wound insertion site.
   Rationale: Reduces the risk of infection.
2 Use transparent sterile occlusive dressings over insertion site.
   Rationale: Permits vision of the wound site.
3 Use dry iodine based spray over the insertion site.
   Rationale: Iodine is an effective antiseptic.
4 Monitor patient's temperature and record.
   Rationale: Permits prompt treatment of infection. If signs of infection arise the catheter may need to be resited.

Problem: Loss of ventricular contraction in response to pacing. (Failure of capture).
Goal: Patient's cardiac output will return to normal.
Nursing Interventions
1 Monitor for signs of shock.
2 Commence resuscitation techniques if ventricular heart rate not sustained.
3 Notify medical staff as soon as possible.
   Rationale: Permits prompt treatment of cardiac arrest.

In certain circumstances the pacemaker misinterprets the information it receives from the heart. The normal heart rate may suddenly reappear, particularly if pacing is used for slow rate arrythmias, or heart block, this intrinsic rate is then in competition with the pacemaker, causing a fast heart rate (tachycardia). Conversely, if the R wave of an intrinsic impulse is not large in amplitude the pacemaker may not sense it and consequently fire off an impulse. This may lead to the dangerous R on T phenomenon. This situation can be rectified by repositioning of the catheter.

If cardiac pacing is instituted, the nurse must precisely and frequently monitor its function and ensure patient safety. Cardio-pulmonary resuscitation must begin immediately if pacing is to sustain the cardiac output. The pacing catheter may stay in situ for several weeks although most dysrhythmias resolve after about ten days. The pacing wire is left in situ for up to one week after dysrhythmias stop, it is then removed.

ATRIOVENTRICULAR HEART BLOCK — EXERCISES

1 What do you understand by the term heart block?
2 What features would you expect to see on the ECG if the heart rhythm were Mobitz Type II?
3 What are the signs and symptoms you would expect with third degree, complete, heart block?
4 How would you recognize an anterior myocardial infarction on a twelve lead ECG?
5 List at least four complications associated with transvenous pacing.
6 What do you understand by the term failure to capture, when discussing transvenous pacing?
7 What do you understand by the term myocardial threshold?
8 What are the differences between syncronized and emergency defibrillation?

4

Monitoring Central Venous Pressure

Central venous pressure monitoring (CVP) is an important tool, as it gives specific information about right sided heart function, venous tone, the return of venous blood flow to the heart and the patient's state of hydration.

In the severely injured or patients who have had major surgery, central venous pressure (CVP) measurement allows prompt recognition of fluid depletion or significant overloading of the circulation, both of which are potentially life threatening conditions. CVP monitoring can detect a reduction in circulating volume before a fall of blood pressure occurs making it of crucial importance in monitoring a critically ill patient.

The circulatory system, (excluding the heart), can be divided into the arterial and venous networks. Although these networks are continuous with each other via the capillary system, for simplicity they will be discussed separately, the venous system in this chapter and the arterial in the next. The veins can be roughly divided into two kinds deep and superficial. The deep veins lie in close proximity to the large arteries and are often called by the same name, i.e. subclavian artery and subclavian vein. The superficial veins lie in the fatty, adipose, tissue just beneath the skin. The superficial and deep veins both carry deoxygenated blood back to the right side of the heart. Monitoring of venous return to the heart therefore gives accurate information about the patient's overall circulatory status.

The veins are composed of three main layers, or coats, which are:

1 The Tunica adventitia, an outer sheath of fibrous tissue.
2 The Tunica media, a middle layer of involuntary muscle fibres and elastic fibrous tissue.
3 The Tunica intima, a lining of endothelium, which provides a smooth inner surface.

The veins are thin walled structures which contain valves. The valves are formed by folds of the lining in the vein and are semi-lunar in appearance. The valves prevent regurgitation of blood backwards into the vein and they therefore assist the venous return of blood to the heart. In some situations the veins become inefficient and are termed varicose, this means that the valves are prevented from closing leading to distention of the veins, this causes unsightly bulging with associated oedema of the feet and legs. Varicose veins are unsightly and cause aching and discomfort in the limbs.

The flow of blood from the veins to the heart is aided by a number of other factors which includes gravity assisted drainage from the upper part of the body and contraction of skeletal muscle, squeezing the veins and pushing the blood onwards towards the heart. During respiration the intra-thoracic pressure changes particularly during inspiration, forces the blood in the great veins to enter the heart.

CENTRAL VENOUS PRESSURE

This is the pressure measured in the great veins, the Superior and Inferior Vena Cavae, it is a reflection of the pressure within the right side of the heart, and indicates how effectively the heart is working as a pump.

The CVP changes very little in normal physiology and is fairly constant within a small range i.e. 0–5 cm of water. Just as a systolic blood pressure reading of 120 mm Hg means that arterial pressure will support a column of mercury 120 mm Hg above the level of the heart, so a CVP reading of 5 cms H_2O means the pressure in the great veins will support a column of water 5 cms above the level of the heart.

It is measured by means of a large bore catheter introduced into one of the larger deep veins. The usual sites for this are the subclavian vein, the brachial vein and in some circumstances the femoral vein. Femoral cannulation is however a less popular choice, due to the increased risks of infection at this insertion site, and the restriction of movement for the patient. Insertion of the cannula is a procedure which must be performed under strict aseptic conditions, because as the cannula is introduced so potentially may infection. Blood is an excellent medium for bacterial growth leading to the risk of septicaemia, a potentially fatal condition.

What Sort of CVP Cannula Should be Used?

There are different reasons for cannulation of a central vein, one of these is measurement of CVP. This procedure rules out the use of certain cannulas which are specifically designed for other uses, some of which may remain in situ for months rather than days. These cannulas i.e. Vygon Nutricath S, are made of a soft silicone coated material and are designed for use in total parentral nutrition (TPN) and should not be used for other purposes such as CVP monitoring. TPN involves the use of special nutritional fluids which often contain glucose and amino acids in high concentration, this makes them vulnerable to bacterial growth. TPN is designed to give a balanced diet containing all the nutritional elements required by the patient however as bacteria have similar gastronomic tastes, these fluids provide an ideal growth medium.

The higher osmolality of TPN fluids makes them highly irritant if given in small peripheral veins, hence the need to give these fluids via a large bore cannula into a central vein. This ensures an adequate blood flow around the cannula to dilute the irritant TPN solution.

The cannulae used for TPN, must be inserted under sterile conditions, using a Seldinger technique. The portion of cannula left outside the skin at the insertion wound site poses a potential infection risk, the catheter is therefore tunnelled beneath the skin, leaving the administration end well away from the insertion site thus reducing the risk of ascending infection. See Figure 4.1 Discussion of the techniques for catheter insertion both for CVP measurement and TPN, can be found on page 85.

A further problem involves the administration of potent

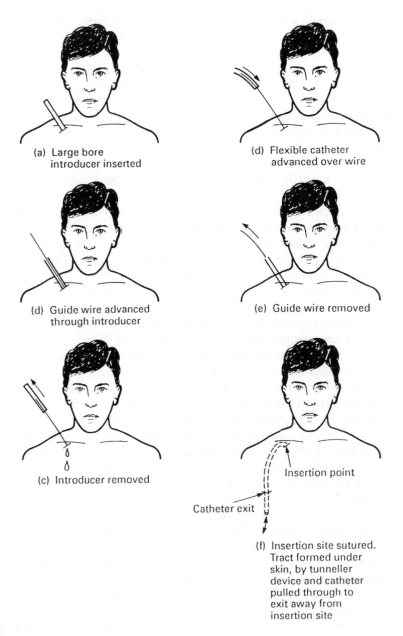

(a) Large bore introducer inserted

(d) Flexible catheter advanced over wire

(d) Guide wire advanced through introducer

(e) Guide wire removed

(c) Introducer removed

Insertion point

Catheter exit

(f) Insertion site sutured. Tract formed under skin, by tunneller device and catheter pulled through to exit away from insertion site

Figure 4.1 *Insertion of subclavian cannula by Seldinger technique.*

drugs that the severely ill patient will usually require to support a failing heart and circulation. These drugs are termed inotropic agents, this means they increase myocardial contraction force and sometimes heart rate. Examples of these drugs are dopamine and adrenaline. The dosage of such drugs tends to be small, often measured in micrograms, and given as number of µg per kilogram of body weight per minute, e.g. 5 µg/Kg/min. The small size of these drug doses and their very potent nature, means that they need to be given as a continuous measured infusion by syringe pump.

The action of these drugs is to increase and support the heart's pumping efficiency by improving the contraction force of the ventricles. Blood pressure is also increased by increasing the peripheral resistance. This also involves shutdown of unnecessary peripheral blood vessels, i.e. those supplying the skin, and diverting the blood to the central area of the body. It is essential these drugs be given into central veins as if they are given into peripheral veins they will be rendered useless as they will become trapped in the vein which will then collapse. The irritancy of these drugs is such that they cause intense pain in the affected limb and may cause necrosis of the vessel and surrounding tissues if blood flow around the cannula is inadequate.

A major hazard associated with use of these drugs in a cannula also used for the manual measurement of CVP is the danger of giving an inadvertent bolus of the drug to the patient. Manual measurement of CVP causes some flushing of the cannula with CVP priming fluid. The connection between the cannula and the administration set usually consists of a three way tap and extension tube. See Figure 4.2.

The extension tube acts as dead space in which the fluid must pass before entering the patient's circulation. When taking a reading the cannula will be flushed by the CVP priming fluid and a bolus of the drug present in the extension tube will be delivered to the patient. **These drugs have a profound effect on the heart and circulation.**

Once the drug has been flushed from the cannula it may take a considerable time for the infusion pump to reprime the dead space. The patient receives no drugs until the dead space is reprimed. The effect of too little/too much of these drugs may be equally lethal. Manual recording of CVP measure-

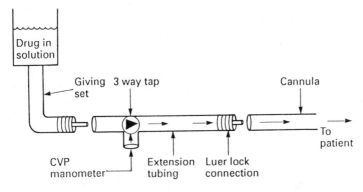

Figure 4.2 Diagram shows the standard arrangement for intravenous infusion and CVP monitoring via CVP cannula.

ments must be carried out using a different central venous catheter to that used when giving TPN or inotropic drugs.

In recent years a variety of cannulas have become available which help to reduce the problem of inadvertent bolus dosage. These cannulas tend to be double or treble lumen, and are in fact two or three separate cannulae fused together. Each cannula having a separate exit point away from the other one or two, i.e. distal, medial, or proximal exit points. This cannula allows concurrent administration of drugs, fluids and CVP measurements. These cannulas are however more expensive than the usual type of cannula, (in some cases up to four or five time the cost).

Other factors taken into consideration prior to cannula selection include special properties of certain cannulas, i.e. silicon and other coating agents which are thought to reduce potential hazard of clot formation, and the medical staff's own experience of inserting catheters they are familar and happy with!

Although the range of cannulae is vast, the insertion technique is largely the same. From the nurse's viewpoint it is important to realize that the size in length and calibre of the catheter is decided by the chosen insertion site and the use the cannula will be put to. The general calibre size of a cannula for an adult is 14 Fg. For subclavian routes the cannulae are approximately 12 inches (30 cms) long. For brachial and femoral cannulation the catheters are 18 inches (45 cms). These cannulae are usually more rigid than those used for TPN. None the less they are flexible enough, to be manipulated through the venous system to a position near the heart. These cannulae, i.e. Wallace Piggy-back catheter or Vygon Leadercath, are inserted using a Seldinger technique. A trocar facilitates entry to the vein and the cannula is then manipulated into position.

PREPARATION OF THE PATIENT

A full explanation of the procedure should be given to the patient. It is important to ensure patient co-operation and confidence, as the procedure can be lengthy if the patient's anatomy is abnormal or if there is patient movement.

It should be explained to the patient that part of the face may be covered with green drapes to prevent contamination of the insertion site and cannula. This can disconcert the patient and it is wise to have a nurse sitting with the patient to reassure him and keep him informed of events. A friendly hand to hold may assist the patient a great deal.

Initially the patient is positioned supine in bed. Warmth and comfort should be assured. Clothing, jewellery and dressings should be removed from the proposed site to prevent risk of contamination and ensure good vision of the site selected.

If the subclavian route is to be used, it will be necessary to position the patient's head down. This causes engorgement of the major veins and prevents any air entering the vein and rising to cause a cerebral embolism.

Preparation of Equipment

Nursing staff will greatly facilitate patient care by ensuring all the equipment is ready promptly. The equipment necessary for the insertion of a CVP cannula is as follows:
1 Sterile gown and gloves.
2 Surgical masks for doctor and assistant
3 Syringes: 5 ml x 1, 10 ml x 2
4 Hypodermic needles: 19g x 2, 21g x 1

5 Lignocaine: 1% or 2%, 5 ml
6 Normal saline: 10 ml
7 Heparin flush solution: 10 units/ml
8 Cleaning solution: e.g. Chlorhexidine in spirit
9 CVP packs containing gallipot, sterile towels, gauze
  swabs, scalpel blade, forceps
10 Suture material: Silk 3/0 or 4/0
11 Needle holder and scissors, (sterile)
12 Extension tube and three-way tap
13 Iodine dry spray
14 Transparent occlusive dressing
15 CVP cannula

Insertion Procedure

Insertion is usually performed by the Seldinger technique. It is
a method of introducing a large bore cannula into a vein
without causing trauma.

The large bore introducer is inserted through the prepared
anaesthetized skin, a small cut with the scalpel blade may be
necessary to facilitate this. The vein is located and punctured,
blood will be seen to flow into the introducer. A flexible wire
with a floppy end then passed through the introducer and
advanced into the vein. The introducer is withdrawn leaving
the wire in place. The wire is designed to cause minimal
trauma to the vein, the floppy end bending rather than
piercing the vein wall. The cannula is then passed over the
wire to the required length and the wire is removed. The
cannula is then connected to the three-way tap and extension
and a rapid blood flow back through the cannula can be
observed, demonstrating correct positioning of the cannula
inside the vein. The cannula is then flushed with heparin
solution to maintain patency and is then sutured in place and
dressed. As can be seen from the description of the technique
above, psychological support is essential for the patient
during this difficult procedure, which is carried out with the
patient fully conscious. Nursing support is therefore vital.

Before use, CVP cannula must be checked for correct
positioning by X-ray. Some catheters can bend back on
themselves, tie in knots, or enter the wrong vessels. Only when

correct positioning of the cannula has been ascertained, can CVP recordings be taken and infusions commenced.

Complications of Insertion

1 Trauma: To the vein or nearby structures. This may cause haemorrhage, pneumo/haemo thorax or haematoma.
2 Pain: If the femoral site is used, there may be damage to the femoral nerve.
3 Pericardial tamponade: Perforation of the pericardium causes haemorrhage within the pericardial sac. The build-up of blood under the pericardium prevents the ventricular muscle from fully expanding at each heart beat and leads to a reduction in cardiac output. This may quickly become serious.

Nursing Role

The potential risks of this procedure make it important to closely monitor the patient following insertion of CVP.

Potential Problem 1: Potential risk of pneumo/haemothorax.
Goal: The patient will have normal respiratory function.
Nursing Interventions
1 Observe respiratory rate and pattern at least every half hour, together with blood pressure and pulse.
   Rationale: Signs and symptoms of pneumothorax do not always appear suddenly, progressive dyspnoea and deterioration of cardio-vascular status may be presenting symptoms.
2 Sit the patient upright in bed, supporting with pillows.
   Rationale: This permits the diaphragm to drop and aids chest expansion. An upright position facilitates the use of accessory muscles of respiration.
3 Give oxygen in high concentration.
   Rationale: This enables adequate arterial oxygen concentration.
4 Have equipment available for insertion of underwater seal drain.
   Rationale: Treatment for this condition is to drain blood or

air from chest and so allow re-expansion of the affected lung.

Potential Problem 2: Shock due to haemorrhage.
Goal: Patient will maintain adequate circulation, with a systolic blood pressure of at least 90 mm Hg. See page 25.

Potential Problem 3: Haematoma over insertion site.
Goal: Haemorrhage will cease.
Nursing Interventions
1 Apply pressure dressing to insertion site.
   Rationale: The object is to prevent extension of haematoma and staunch blood flow.
2 Observe for signs of extending haematoma.
   Rationale: These may indicate internal haemorrhage.
3 Inform medical staff.

Problem 4: Pain at insertion site.
Goal: Patient will not experience pain.
Nursing Interventions
1 Observe insertion site for signs of bruising, haematoma and swelling.
   Rationale: This is to achieve early detection of signs of infection of haematoma and swelling.
2 Adjust dressings for patient comfort.
3 Give prescribed analgesia.
4 Inform and record findings of wound inspection to medical staff.

Potential Problem 5: Risk of cardiac tamponade.
Goal: Patient will maintain sufficient cardiac function to sustain life.
Nursing Interventions
1 Carry out nursing intervention as for shock
   Rationale: Cardiac tamponade reduces cardiac output and may lead to ventricular dysrhythmia.
2 Obtain medical assistance.
3 Prepare patient for surgery in accordance with hospital protocols.
   Rationale: Emergency cardiac surgery and relief of tampo-

nade will be necessary. Speed is of the essence in this potentially lethal situation.

MANUAL CVP MEASUREMENT (INTERMITTENT)

In the ward situation it will be necessary to take intermittent measurements of the CVP. This procedure is becoming a more commonly used technique. In the surgical ward it is an accurate method of assessing the circulating volume and right sided heart pressure. This is particularly helpful when caring for the post operative patient. It allows prompt replacement of fluid without the danger of overloading the circulation and increasing heart workload.

Equipment

1 Intravenous administration set.
2 Prescribed bag of infusion: (5% Dextrose, 0.9% Saline), although 0.9% Saline may be contra-indicated in some situations. Plasma or plasma expanders, i.e. dextran, Gelofusine and Haemacel must not be used for CVP measurement, nor should any fluids of high osmolarity. 0.9% saline may be contra-indicated in patients suffering from renal failure with associated hypernatraemia, or intractable pulmonary oedema. CVP readings are expressed as centimetres of water, the high specific gravity of solutions such as Haemacel or 50% dextrose means any reading obtained will be very different from that obtained with water, dextrose or saline, which have a similar specific gravity to water.
3 CVP manometer set.
4 Spirit level.

Central Venous Pressure can be Measured in Several Ways

Direct measurement involves connection of a manometer tube to a cannula situated in the central veins. See Figure 4.3. The pressure present in the large veins is transmitted through the tubing to fluid inside the manometer. The fluid level will rise or fall with the pressure in the veins. This is the Central Venous Pressure, (CVP).

Respiratory movements change the intrathoracic pressure, consequently the fluid level in the manometer will fluctuate with respiration. The CVP reading will be the height of a column of water that can be supported by the pressure in the vein.

To ensure accurate readings are taken the zero point should first be decided. This is important because all the readings must be made from the same zero.

The true zero point is situated just outside the right atria at the level of the Vena Cavae. In practice however a more conveniently measured zero point is used, unfortunately there are two such reference points in common usage which may lead to confusion.

The first zero point is the Angle of Louis, this is the sternal notch, located in the centre of the chest at the third intercostal space. The second and more commonly used point is the fifth intercostal space in the mid-axillary line.

Either of these points can be used but they are not interchangeable. The nurse must use the same point consistently to ensure measurements are made from the same baseline. The position of the patient is important. If the patient is level for the first reading, all subsequent readings must be taken with the patient level, or if the patient is lying at an angle, all subsequent readings must be taken with the patient lying at the same angle. This is to ensure consistency so that any changes that occur are real changes in the patient's condition, not due to changes in procedure.

PROCEDURE FOR MANUAL CVP MONITORING

1 Prepare the equipment.
   • Connect administration set to infusion and prime the set.
   • Connect the administration set to the CVP manometer.
   • Ensure all air bubbles are removed from the system.
   Rationale: This is to prevent air embolism.
2 Connect the system to the CVP cannula.
3 Attach the manometer set to the infusion stand.
4 Locate the position of zero reference point, mid-axillary

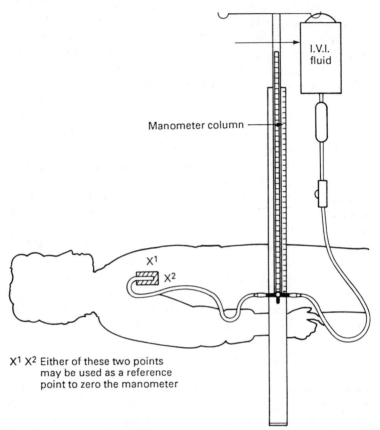

I.V.I.
fluid

Manometer column ⏤

X¹

X²

X¹ X² Either of these two points
    may be used as a reference
    point to zero the manometer

Figure 4.3 *Direct central venous pressure measurement.*

line fifth intercostal space. Position the 0 on the manometer
column in a horizontal line with the reference point on the
patient's skin. Use the spirit level to ensure this is done
exactly.
Rationale: This establishes the baseline and ensures accuracy of readings.
5 Fill the manometer:
  • Turn the manometer three-way tap 'OFF' to the patient,
    and 'ON' to the giving set. See Figure 4.4.
  • Fill the manometer up to +/−20 cm of intravenous fluid,
    but no further.
    Rationale: The manometer is open to the atmosphere,

cotton filters in the manometer prevent contamination by bacteria, but these become useless if wet.

6 Take the CVP measurement:
- Turn the three-way tap 'OFF' to infusion 'ON' to the manometer and CVP cannula.
- Observe the fluid level in the manometer, and note fluctuations, due to respiration.
  Rationale: Changes in the fluid level due to respiration are normal—the fluid in the manometer will fall rapidly at first, then slowly reach the correct level.
7 Observe and record measurement.
8 Recommence infusion (To maintain patency of CVP cannula.):
- Turn three-way tap 'OFF' to the manometer, and 'ON' to the patient and infusion set.
- Regulate infusion rate.
9 Observe CVP recordings hourly, or as prescribed.
Rationale: Serial recordings show trends which will permit prompt treatment of dehydration (hypovolaemia), or overloading of the circulation.

CVP Monitoring Using a Pressure Monitor

Direct continuous CVP measurements, using a pressure monitor, permits close observation of the trends in CVP pressure in the seriously ill patient. This method is similar to a direct measurement technique, but the readings are transmitted from a transducer to a monitor.

A transducer converts physical pressure into an electrical signal which is relayed to a monitor where it is displayed as a digital reading and a waveform pattern. This process is similar to ECG measurement, where signals from a rate meter are displayed on a monitor.

The transducer is usually a flat metal plate which acts as a strain gauge. Fitted over the plate is a plastic disc, or dome, which is rigid on one side and flexible on the other. It is primed with fluid and connected to the CVP cannula. The venous pressure is transmitted to the dome through the tubing and causes the disc to bulge on the flexible side which in turn causes pressure on the transducer plate. This is sensed and

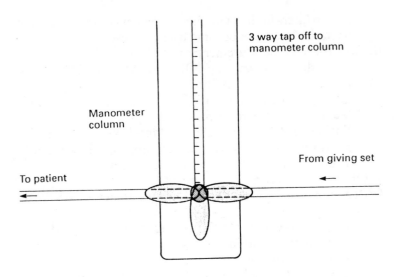

3 way tap off to
manometer column

Manometer
column

From giving set

To patient

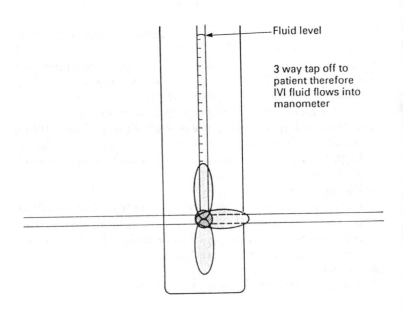

Fluid level

3 way tap off to
patient therefore
IVI fluid flows into
manometer

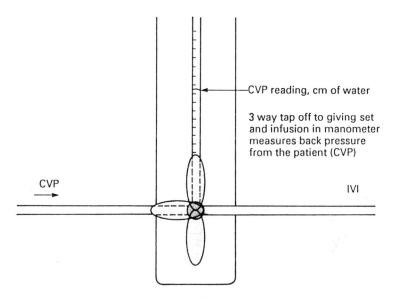

Figure 4.4   *CVP measurement using a water manometer.*

transmitted as an electrical signal to the monitor, where it is displayed. See Figure 4.5.

PREPARATION FOR DIRECT CVP MEASUREMENT

Equipment

For situations where set-ups are not pre-assembled:
1 Pressure transducer dome (sterile disposable).
2 500 ml Hartmann's Solution (used because pH is nearer to blood pH than other solutions).
3 Heparin, 1000 units (without bacteriocide or preservative as this is less of an irritant).
4 Pressure bag or pump.
5 Intra flow device (permits 3 ml per hour of flush solution to enter the cannula from the bag, also can permit continuous fast flushing of the cannula with fluid under pressure from an infusion bag).
6 Giving set.
7 150 cm length of high pressure tubing.

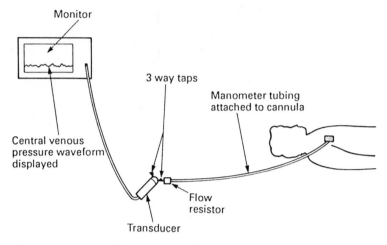

Figure 4.5 *Central venous pressure monitor.*

8 Three-way taps x 2.
9 10 ml syringe.
10 1 ml syringe.

Method

See Figure 4.6.
1 Prepare transducer:
  ● Remove transducer from static holder.
  ● Place a few drops of sterile water onto transducer plate.
    Rationale: This ensures contact with dome—use water as saline may cause damage to the transducer plate. Refer to manufacturer's instruction manual, certain transducers do not require the use of water between the dome and plate to improve contact.
  ● Remove sterile dome from pack, attach to transducer plate, leave end caps on dome in place.
    Rationale: This prevents contamination of the dome.
2 Replace transducer on to the holder.
3 Switch on the monitor and connect transducers.
4 Prepare heparinized Hartmann's solution:
  ● Add the heparin to the Hartmann's solution.
  ● Connect the giving set to the infusion bag ensuring that the clamps are turned off.

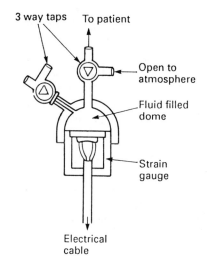

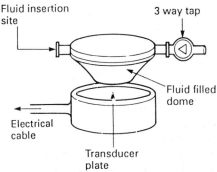

Figure 4.6 *Diagram showing two types of pressure transducers and domes.*

5 Attach the pressure bag or pump over the infusion bag and increase pressure to 50 mm Hg.
   Rationale: The pressure must be higher than the central venous pressure to prevent backflow of blood into the transducer.
6 Prime the Administration Set, intraflow and high pressure tubing by:
   • Attaching the three-way tap to the female connector of the intraflow. Turn the tap 'OFF' to the intraflow.
   • Connect the high pressure tubing to the male connector of the pressure resistor, intraflow (see Figure 4.7).

- Attach the giving set to the long line port of the intraflow (see Figure 4.7).
- Attach the 10 ml syringe to the three-way tap between the intraflow and the transducer.
- Turn the three-way tap 'ON' to the intraflow, and 'OFF' to the transducer. Pull the intraflow tab and fill the syringe with the flush solution.
- Turn the three-way tap 'OFF' to the intraflow and 'ON' to the transducer.
- Open the IV clamp and pull on the intraflow tab to prime the assembled set up. Ensure all air bubbles are removed from the system.
  Rationale: This ensures accurate pressure measurement and reduces 'damping' of the trace and the risk of air embolism.
- Remove the end cap from the exposed dome port.
  Rationale: This vents the transducer to air.
- Flush the transducer using the pre-filled syringe, ensuring all air bubbles are removed.
- Close the end cap over the exposed port of the dome.
  Rationale: This turns the transducer 'OFF' to air.
- Remove the syringe and replace all end caps.
  Rationale: This maintains a closed system and reduces risk of contamination.
7 Check zero calibration.
   - Turn the three-way tap 'OFF' to the intraflow.
   - Remove the sterile cap from the three-way tap port.
     Rationale: This vents the transducer to air.
   - Check the zero calibration of the monitor according to the manufacturer's instructions. This usually entails pressing the zero button for 2–3 seconds with the transducer vented to air. The digital reading on the pressure monitor should return to zero.
     Rationale: The transducer must be balanced/calibrated to room temperature giving a zero reading to ensure accuracy of measurement.
8 Commence continuous CVP readings.
   - Turn the three-way tap 'ON' to the intraflow and the transducer.
   - Replace the sterile cap to the three-way tap.
   - Position the transducer level with the skin zero reference

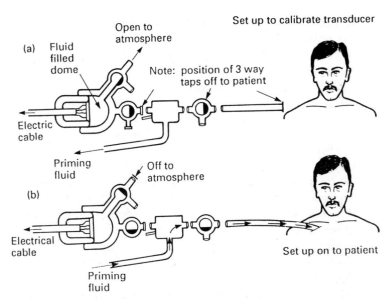

Figure 4.7 *Diagram showing how the equipment is arranged for monitoring pressure.*

point, either the fifth intercostal space, mid-axillary line, or the angle of Louis. Check the position with a spirit level.

Rationale: This ensures accurate readings because, for every 2.5 cm the transducer is lower than the skin reference point, the reading on the monitor is 2 mm Hg higher than the actual CVP.

NURSING INTERVENTIONS AND RATIONALES

1 Strict aseptic technique is vital during preparation of the system. This is of equal importance for both the indirect and direct methods of CVP monitoring.
   Rationale: Cannulation of the veins permits direct access by bacteria into the blood stream, through contamination of the cannula, administration sets, fluids, and the wound site.
2 The patency of the CVP cannula must be maintained at all times.

Rationale: This is a potentially hazardous procedure for the patient. Insertion of the cannula also involves some discomfort. Patient safety is paramount – embolization from clots formed in the cannula are potentially lethal. Recannulation of the veins and the inherent risks must not be taken lightly.

3 Ensure that all connections are secure, and that the number of connectors, three-way taps etc., are kept to a minimum.

Rationale: This reduces the optional risk of haemorrhage, air embolism, inaccurate recordings and contamination by bacteria. All connectors should have luer lock capability – this reduces the risk of accidental disconnection.

4 Observe and record vital signs frequently.

Rationale: Local infection of the wound site may be readily apparent, septicaemia may not. Pyrexia, tachycardia and some degree of hypertension may herald sepsis. Signs of shock may also be present due to septicaemia, haemorrhage or embolism.

5 Redress the wound, usually only if required, i.e. if the dressing is moist or soiled.

Rationale: Transparent occlusive dressings permit direct inspection of the wound site without disturbance to the dressing. If the wound is dry and clean the dressing should be left in position. The use of dry povidone spray over the cannula entry site reduces the risk of infection.

6 Observe CVP for significant changes and report.

Rationale: Using the direct method of measurement, poor fluid oscillation in the manometer, or inadequate flow of fluid through the cannula may indicate that the cannula is obstructed. This may be a potential cause of embolus formation.

Using the indirect method of measurement, change in the waveform on the monitor, or reduction in the rate of flow of fluid through the cannula may be due to cannula obstruction.

7 Change the monitoring tubing to the cannula every 24 hours.

Rationale: This reduces the risk of contamination by bacteria.

8 Check the transducer/monitor position against the skin

reference point before each reading and after each change in patient position.

Rationale: This ensures accuracy of measurements. Some units attach the transducer to the patient.

9 Ensure the tubing and cables are not kinked or dragging.

10 Ensure the pressure bag is inflated to 50 mm Hg at all times.

Rationale: This prevents backflow of blood into the transducer and so prevents inaccurate measurements and wastage of expensive equipment.

11 Observe for cardiac dysrhythmias.

Rationale: A venous cannulae can move and be drawn into the right ventricle where they cause irritation and dysrhythmias.

12 Venous pressure readings taken on an artificially ventilated patient give falsely high readings.

Rationale: Artificial ventilation causes intermittent positive pressure within the thorax during inspiration. This causes the readings to be artificially high. Most units have policies which acknowledge that IPPV causes false CVP readings and make appropriate allowance for this. A figure of 5 cm is usual, this figure being deducted from the CVP recording to give a truer reading, i.e. if the CVP is 20 cm and 5 cm is subtracted from this reading the CVP will be 15 cms.

REMOVAL OF A CVP CANNULA

To remove a CVP cannula, the suture holding it in place needs to be cut. The cannula is withdrawn slowly and the nurse should observe for the ease of withdrawal and note any resistance or patient discomfort. In either case, secure the cannula and seek medical assistance. The cannula length should be checked to ensure it is intact as a cannula may fracture leading to embolization. Without touching the cannula except with forceps, place the tip in a culture medium. A pressure dressing would then be applied. While some bleeding from the insertion site is usual, delayed haemorrhage must be prevented.

Complications of CVP Monitoring and Cannulation

1 Haemorrhage
2 Sepsis
3 Air emboli
4 Cannula fracture
5 Phlebitis
6 Vein trauma
7 Pneumothorax
8 Dysrhythmia
9 Altered skin integrity.

Conclusion

CVP measurements give important information about the right heart pressure, venous tone and venous return, accurate recording permits the early treatment of serious fluid imbalance. The potential hazards for the patient, however, are numerous, and it is vital that the nurse is fully conversant with the technique before carrying it out.

MONITORING CENTRAL VENOUS PRESSURE — EXERCISES

1 List three situations where CVP monitoring would be advantageous.
2 What information can be obtained from CVP measurement?
3 Where are the usual CVP cannula insertion sites?
4 Describe the nursing interventions necessary during insertion.
5 What are the hazards of CVP cannulation to the patient?
6 Briefly describe the procedure for measuring the CVP by the direct method.
7 Where on the body are the zero reference points?
8 Describe what observations you would make when caring for a patient with a CVP cannula.
9 List the complications of CVP monitoring and cannulation.
10 What are the normal values (range) of central venous pressure?

5

Arterial Pressure Monitoring

Direct arterial pressure monitoring has become a more common sight in the Intensive Unit. This method of monitoring is usually more accurate than manual recordings taken with a sphygmomanometer, although it has many inherent hazards for the patient. Blood pressure measurement is an important technique in three ways – it helps to confirm medical diagnosis, determines treatment and monitors response to therapy. Arterial pressure monitoring primarily gives information about left heart function and the haemodynamic state of the patient.

Before discussion of the arterial blood pressure monitoring technique, the normal anatomy and physiology of the arterial network needs to be recalled.

ARTERIAL NETWORK

Arteries and arterioles vary considerably in size but their structure is similar. The arterial vessels, like the veins are composed of three layers:
1 The Tunica adventitia, an outer fibrous sheath.
2 The Tunica media, a coat of elastic and involuntary muscle fibres. In the large arteries this layer has more elastic tissue than muscle fibres. This coat is much thicker than that found in the veins, probably due to the higher pressure the arteries have to cope with.
3 The Tunica intima, an inner lining of smooth flattened squamous epithelium. The smooth surface of this layer

reduces the risk of formation and prevents turbulent blood flow through the artery.

As the arterial network divides, the final link between the arterial and venous systems merge is the capillary. Unlike arteries and arterioles, capillaries are minute vessels composed of a single layer of cells. The diameter of the vessel is therefore small but wide enough to allow the passage of red blood cells.

The arterial system is supplied with oxygenated blood from the left side of the heart which it transports to the tissues. After the delivery of oxygen and nutrients in exchange for waste products of metabolism, the deoxygenated blood is returned to the right side of the heart via the venous system.

Nerve Input

Arterial blood vessels receive sympathetic nervous input to the muscle lining which maintains them in a state of constrictor tone, see section on blood pressure.

Blood Pressure

Following ventricular contraction, blood flows through the arterial network from a region of high pressure to a region of low pressure. The arteries are always in tone, which means the muscle coat never fully relaxes.

The first determinant of arterial blood pressure is the amount of blood pumped into the arterial system, this is known as the cardiac output. At each contraction the two ventricles of the heart expel approximately 70 ml of blood each, this is termed the stroke volume.

The ventricular contraction phase is termed systole, and the ventricular relaxation phase diastole. The systolic blood pressure indicates the maximum pressure produced by the left ventricle during systole. The diastolic pressure is the pressure in the artery at the end of diastole. Pressures measured in the left ventricle would be approximately 120 mm Hg at systole, and 7–8 mm Hg at diastole. In the aorta, however, the effect of constrictor tone helps maintain the diastolic pressure at around 70–80 mm Hg.

The other key factor in maintaining blood pressure is the peripheral resistance offered by the network of arterioles throughout the body. The diameter of the arterioles determines the amount of resistance offered. If the arteriole is constricted due to sympathetic nerve activity then peripheral resistance will increase. Conversely, relaxation of the muscle layer in the wall of the arteriole causes the diameter of the vessel to increase, thus reducing peripheral resistance.

Changes in peripheral resistance can cause dramatic changes in arterial blood pressure. This can be seen in hypothermic patients where generalized shutdown of peripheral vessels will have occurred to conserve heat and maintain the circulation to the heart and brain. Sudden warming will induce peripheral dilation which in turn will cause the blood pressure to fall dramatically.

Regulation of Arterial Tone

Regulation of arterial tone is controlled by the vaso-motor centre in the medulla of the brain. The vaso-motor centre (VMC) receives information concerning blood pressure from the baroreceptors in the carotid bodies and the arch of aorta. This information determines the activity of the VMC. If the blood pressure falls then the baroreceptor signals to the VMC are reduced and the VMC responds by increasing sympathetic tone in the arterioles causing them to constrict increasing peripheral resistance and therefore increasing blood pressure. Conversely, a high blood pressure stimulates the baroreceptors to discharge frequent signals to the VMC, which then reduces the sympathetic tone allowing the arterioles to dilate, reducing the peripheral resistance to help maintain blood pressure at a more normal level (see Figure 5.1). This feedback system maintains a nearly constant level of blood pressure and helps the body compensate for the different forms of stress it may be exposed to. Other mechanisms affecting the vaso-motor centre and arteriole vessel size are as follows:

Carbon Dioxide

Excess carbon dioxide causes increased VMC activity and therefore increased peripheral resistance. A low carbon dioxide level has the opposite effect.

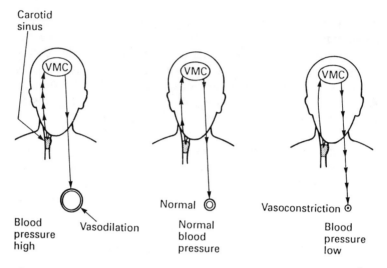

Figure 5.1 *Baroreceptor and vasomotor centre (VMC)* ✦ *activity and arteriolar tone.*

Oxygen
Lack of oxygen causes increased VMC activity, and therefore raised blood pressure due to increased peripheral resistance.

Stress, Emotion and Pain
Stress, emotional upset and pain increase VMC activity and raise blood pressure by increasing peripheral resistance. Catecholamines released in response to stress, i.e. adrenaline and noradrenaline, increase sympathetic nerve activity and add to the effects of VMC activity, that is, increased peripheral resistance and thus increased blood pressure.

Blood Viscosity
Changes in packed cell volume affect viscosity and hence alter peripheral resistance.

Renin, Angiotensin
Renin is an enzyme indirectly involved in the control of blood vessel size. It is released when blood flow to the kidneys is reduced. It acts on a substrate from the liver to form angiotensinogen, which is converted to angiotensin. Angiotensin is a powerful vaso-constrictor which increases blood pressure.

Exercise
During exercise there will be an increase in the waste products

of metabolism. Blood flow to the muscles is increased, not only to provide adequate oxygen and nutrients, but also to remove the waste products.

Heat and Cold

A cold environment leads to peripheral vasoconstriction, while dilation occurs in a warm environment.

Cardiac Output

Cardiac output is a main determining factor in the maintenance of blood pressure, but is not totally reliant on peripheral resistance – changes in peripheral resistance cause changes in blood pressure rather than directly affecting cardiac output.

METHODS OF ASSESSING BLOOD PRESSURE

The methods employed to measure blood pressure fall into two groups, indirect and direct recording.

Indirect Methods

Sphygmomanometer

The most common and familiar method of measuring blood pressure is by sphygmomanometer. This technique demands careful attention to detail as the most common cause of inaccuracy is due to operator error. To avoid error the size of the cuff must be correct, i.e. it should extend at least one and a half turns around the arm. Too small or too large a cuff causes inaccurate readings. The patient should be sitting or lying, and be relaxed as anxiety will produce a falsely high reading. The upper arm should be exposed, with the sleeve rolled back in such a way as not to be tight around the arm. The tubes to the cuff must not be twisted or kinked, and the sphygmomanometer must be at the same level as the patient's heart for an accurate reading. The position of the brachial artery can be confirmed by palpation. The cuff is inflated to 200 mm Hg to compress the artery and a stethoscope is quickly placed over the brachial artery to check that no pulse is discernable. If so, the valve of the pump is unscrewed and the pressure slowly released at approximately 3–5 mm Hg at a time. Eventually a feint tapping sound will be heard, (as the blood is being forced into the limb). This is the **systolic pressure.**

The explanation of this phenomenon is quite simple. At systolic blood pressure the blood can just force its way into the artery. As it does so, the flow is turbulent and it is the sound of this turbulent blood flow that you can hear through the stethoscope. The tapping sounds will increase to a loud knocking noise, the sound of blood entering the artery during systole only.

As the cuff pressure continues to fall the sounds become abruptly muffled, this is the **diastolic pressure.** Shortly after this the sounds disappear. This indicates blood flow has returned to the normal laminar or smooth flow that usually exists in the arterial system, such a flow is silent. These sounds, heard when recording blood pressure in this way, are termed Korotkoff sounds, after their discoverer.

Automatic Blood Pressure Monitoring

At present there are a number of devices available for automatic cuff pressure recording. They generally involve attaching a cuff to the patient's arm and selecting an automatic mode switch. These machines are designed to measure non-invasively and automatically systolic and diastolic pressure, mean arterial pressure and pulse rate. They can be used for neonatal, paediatric and adult patients. A microprocessor within the machine rejects artifact from other electrical equipment and patient movement. Once inflated to 180 mm Hg the monitor begins a stepped deflation until systole is identified, deflation then continues until the mean arterial blood pressure (diastolic) and pulse are recorded. The results of the recordings are displayed as a digital read-out. The monitor can be preset to take recordings at timed intervals from one to sixty minutes.

Disadvantages of Indirect Blood Pressure Measurement

1 Frequent blood pressure recordings involve discomfort and even pain for the patient. For the seriously ill patient, this can be very tiresome and adds to their anxiety and distress.

2 The patient's awareness of blood pressure measurement will often give a falsely high reading for the reasons explained above.

3 Inaccuracies in recording may be caused by incorrect cuff size in relation to the patient's limb.

4 Portable sphygmomanometers may become inaccurate due to excessive movement and rough handling, and they therefore must be checked and re-calibrated regularly.

5 The cuff and tubing are made from a rubberized material which eventually perishes causing cracking and hence inaccuracies in readings.

6 The cuff method establishes the systolic pressure from approximately one cardiac contraction, thus an isolated weak contraction, e.g. due to a ventricular ectopic, will give an artificially low reading.

7 There is scope for a wide range of operator error due to factors such as poor technique or different hearing acuity.

Direct Blood Pressure Measurement

Direct blood pressure readings permit continuous monitoring of blood pressure. This may be vital for the early treatment of hypovolaemia as in certain situations arterial blood pressure may fall before the central venous pressure. Patients receiving potent anti-hypertensive agents via an intravenous line may also benefit from continuous blood pressure monitoring. The technique, however, has many hazards associated with it and should not be taken lightly.

Arterial monitoring is carried out by inserting a cannula into a peripheral artery, usually the radial artery, although the brachial, femoral and dorsalis pedis arteries may also be used. (See Figure 5.2). The radial artery is favoured because, although it restricts movement to some extent, the patient, with care, can still use the affected limb, and the wrist and hand usually have a good collateral circulation. In addition, the artery lies close to the surface and in most cases is somewhat easier to cannulate.

Before insertion of the cannula the doctor should check that an adequate collateral circulation exists. This is achieved by performing Allen's Test.

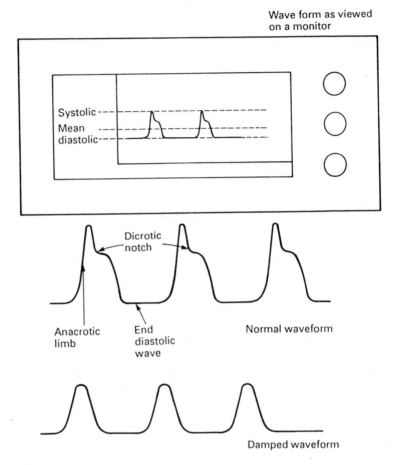

Wave form as viewed on a monitor

Systolic

Mean

diastolic

Dicrotic notch

Anacrotic limb

End diastolic wave

Normal waveform

Damped waveform

Figure 5.2 *Pressure waveforms.*

Allen's Test

The radial and ulnar arteries are located in the limb and are occluded by pressure. The patient is asked to flex the fingers, which should then cause the hand to blanche. Pressure is maintained on the radial artery and released from the ulnar. If the ulnar circulation is adequate, the hand should flush indicating good capillary flow. If the ulnar circulation is inadequate, cannulation of the radial artery should not be performed as the hand will not have an adequate alternative blood supply.

A similar test can be performed on the lower leg by occluding the posterior tibial and the dorsalis pedis arteries. When the foot blanches, the posterior tibial artery pressure is released and capillary flushing is taken to indicate adequate collateral blood flow.

PREPARATION FOR INSERTION OF ARTERIAL CANNULA

Equipment

1 Arterial parallel sided cannula, (size 20–22 for an adult)
2 Pack with swabs, gallipot and forceps
3 Chlorhexidine Spirit lotion, skin preparation
4 Suture material
5 Needle holder
6 Dry iodine spray
7 Lignocaine injection ampoule, 2 ml
8 2 ml syringe
9 Hypodermic needle
10 Transparent occlusive dressing
11 High pressure tubing, (must be high pressure tubing, ordinary flexible tubing is too compliant and causes inaccurate measurement)
12 Three-way tap
13 Flush solution (heparinized Hartmann's)

Procedure

The procedure must be fully explained to the patient to gain patient co-operation and prevent dislodging of the cannula and to reduce patient anxiety. The patient is positioned comfortably in bed with the arm supported on a pillow. The artery may be cannulated by the Seldinger Technique, as for CVP cannulation, or by trocar and cannula.

Insertion by the Seldinger Technique

The large bore introducer is inserted through the prepared anaesthetized skin, a small cut with the scalpel blade may be necessary to facilitate this. The artery is located and punctured, blood will be seen to flow into the introducer. A flexible wire with a floppy end is then passed through the introducer and advanced into the artery. The introducer is withdrawn leaving the wire in place. The wire is designed to cause minimal trauma to the artery, the floppy end bending rather than piercing the artery wall. The cannula is then passed over the wire to the required length and the wire is removed (see Figure 4.1). The cannula is then connected to the three-way tap and extension and rapid blood flow back through the cannula can be observed, this demonstrates correct positioning of the cannula inside the artery. The cannula is then flushed with the heparin solution to maintain potency and the cannula is then sutured in place and dressed.

The transducer dome measures the pressure in the artery and the transducer then converts this to a small electrical current which can be amplified and displayed on a monitor. This is a very delicate and sensitive piece of electronic equipment which can provide vital information when treated correctly, but if treated incorrectly it can provide inaccurate information extremely easily!

The function of the arterial catheter and three-way tap is to permit access to the patient's arteries for blood sampling and to transfer the hydraulic pressure (blood pressure) detected at the catheter tip, to the transducer dome. The waveform seen on the monitor consists of a sharp rapid upstroke, the anacrotic limb, a defined dicrotic notch and the end diastolic wave (see Figure 5.2).

TROUBLESHOOTING

1 Resonance

The fluid within the transducer set-up can resonate (oscillate). This resonance has its own characteristic frequency and can distort the trace on the monitor, causing higher readings than actually exist. This may be particularly true in patients who have pathological or drug induced hypertension, i.e. the greater the haemodynamic energy applied, the greater the oscillations within the equipment. Reduction of the resonance can be achieved only when the blood pressure is reduced to a more normal level.

It is good practice to measure the blood pressure by the indirect method at least once per shift, to check the accuracy of the direct electrical monitoring equipment.

2 Damping

The monitoring equipment responds readily to any changes in pressure. This sensitivity is compensated by the equipment with a mechanism known as damping. However, other factors can cause further damping leading to distortion of the waveform and inaccurate measurement (see Figure 5.3). The presence of air bubbles is one example as well as posing a potential risk of air embolism. The transducer dome and the three-way tap are the most likely areas where air may become trapped, although the whole set-up is vulnerable. Careful priming will reduce the incidence of air bubbles.

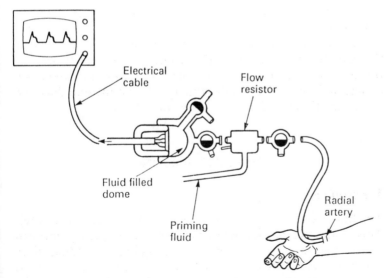

Figure 5.3   *Diagram showing the arrangement of equipment for monitoring pressure. Refer to Figure 4.7 (a) substitute an arm (as above) for the patient.*

Kinking of the cannula, or poor positioning of the cannula within the artery will also cause damping. Careful observation, secure dressings, and suturing of the cannula in situ, will help to prevent this.

3 Blood in the Equipment

The presence of blood within the equipment, particularly in the transducer dome, will distort the trace. This problem is normally due to operator error. It is emphasized that careful monitoring, correct alarm settings and observations of patient response are imperative. The tube connections must be secure and the flush solution must be pressurized to a level greater than the systolic pressure to prevent back tracking of the blood into the equipment, or onto the floor. Always remember this equipment has been introduced into a major artery, consequently incorrect positioning of the three-way tap can cause significant haemorrhage.

Other causes of a distorted or inaccurate measurement include:
- Transducer position. They should be placed near to or at the same level as the heart.
  Too high, and a false low reading is displayed.
  Too low, and a false high reading is displayed.
- Use of excessively long tubing reduces the frequency response of the set-up making it less sensitive. Pressure changes may not be detected or displayed on the monitor, as a result, the dicrotic notch may become poorly defined. The use of too long tubing also increases the risk of air bubbles being trapped in the tubing, usually at luer lock connections.

- The transducer is also affected by changes in environmental temperature. It is therefore good practice to calibrate the transducer at least once per shift to ensure accuracy.
- Rough handling of the transducer can alter the calibration, so always handle with care.
- In addition to transducers, monitors can also go wrong. Frequent checks, according to the manufacturer's instructions are necessary to ensure accuracy.

HAZARDS TO THE PATIENT

As has been already stated, cannulation of arteries has many inherent hazards for the patient, these include:

Potential Risk of Haemorrhage Haemotoma
Goal: The limb will have an adequate circulation and haemorrhage will not occur.
Nursing Intervention
1 Ensure the cannula site is visible and not covered by bed linen or night clothes. It is preferable to place the limb against a white background.
2 Dress the cannula site with transparent occlusive dressing.
3 Identify with red tape.
   Rationale: Blood viewed against a white sheet, is instantly recognizable and eye catching. If the cannula site is obscured, accidental de-cannulation or disconnection may not be apparent for some time, particularly if the high/low alarms have been switched off.

Haemorrhage
Goal: Haemorrhage will cease as soon as possible if it does occur.
Nursing Intervention
1 Apply direct pressure over the bleeding site.
2 Check the security of the tube connections.
3 Ensure the three-way taps are correctly positioned.
4 Ensure the flush container is pressurized to 200 mm Hg.
5 Inform doctor.
6 If haemorrhage persists, turn the set-up off and apply a pressure dressing over the site. Remain with the patient until medical assistance arrives.

Sepsis at Cannula Site
Goal: No sepsis will occur.
Nursing Intervention
1 Ensure the cannulation and set-up are prepared and performed under aseptic conditions.
2 Ensure all entry points are filled with sterile stoppers.
3 Perform all dressings using strict aseptic technique.
4 Change equipment as per hospital policy.

Rationale: Change of set-up varies from hospital to hospital, although every 24 hours is recommended.

Potential Risk of Embolization
Goal: Prevent embolization (reduce risk).
Nursing Intervention
1 Check the integrity of all connections.
2 Ensure the flush solution is at a pressure of 300 mm Hg and ensure the level of solution in the bag is adequate and air free.
3 Ensure careful priming of the set-up, as bubbles of air can become lodged.

Spasm of the Artery
Goal: Arterial spasm will not occur.
Nursing Intervention
1 Ensure the flush solution is at room temperature.
2 Do not flush the cannula excessively.
   Rationale: Cold fluid under pressure will cause arterial spasm with the associated risk of thrombus formation and pain. Excessive flushing has a similar effect, causing a potential risk of skin necrosis, ischaemia, thrombosis and gangrene. Arterial cannulation should not be used for longer than seven days. Rotation of arterial cannulation sites may be necessary if arterial monitoring is required for a prolonged period.

Inadequate Blood Flow due to Arterial Spasm as shown by Blanching and Pain
Goal: Adequate circulation to limb.
Nursing Intervention
1 Request arterial line is removed.
2 Observe the circulation to hand and fingers closely and report findings.
3 Do not flush the cannula.
4 Keep the limb warm.
   Rationale: Warmth promotes capillary dilation. In some cases, ganglion block with drugs may be necessary to decrease sympathetic nerve activity to the artery thus reducing spasm. The cannula should always be removed.

Potential Risk of Thrombus Formation
Goal: Thrombus formation will not occur.
Nursing Intervention
1 Ensure the flush solution is pressurized to 300 mm Hg.
2 Ensure adequate flush solution is in the set-up.
3 Ensure 1,000 units of heparin has been added to the flush solution, thus preventing thrombus formation within the catheter.
4 Prevent excessive movement of the cannula.
   Rationale: This is to prevent formation of thrombus and reduces the risk of embolization.

Within the Intensive Care and Coronary Care units, direct arterial monitoring is convenient and relatively easy to use. It enables prompt treatment of potential life threatening situations and allows the seriously ill patient to rest without frequent disturbances and discomfort.

The hazards however are many, and it is vital that set-up and subsequent care is meticulous. Permanent damage to the hand is possible and can result in a wide range of consequences for the patient. These may include loss of independence and employment, and permanent disability and pain.

If we are to be able to help and not harm our patients, we must ensure that we understand the implications of the procedure, and give appropriate efficient care.

ARTERIAL PRESSURE MONITORING — EXERCISES

1 Give three reasons for measuring a patient's blood pressure.
2 What do you understand by the term 'peripheral resistance'?
3 What factors are involved in the regulation of blood vessel calibre/diameter?
4 Describe, as you would to a student nurse, how you would measure blood pressure by the indirect method.
5 What are Korotkoff sounds?
6 Give three sources of error in indirect blood pressure recordings.

7 In what situations would direct blood pressure monitoring be used?
8 Describe Allen's Test.
9 Describe how a transducer works.
10 List the hazards of arterial cannulation.

6

Swan Ganz Monitoring

We have seen how continual accurate monitoring of the patient's cardiovascular status is crucial in high dependency settings. A further method of obtaining this information involves the use of a Swan Ganz catheter. This is a special catheter which has a small inflatable balloon at its end which is inserted into a large vein and floated through the right side of the heart and up into the pulmonary artery. The catheter, can be attached to a transducer to allow monitoring of pressure changes within each part of the heart. This information can be recorded and displayed to assist in the diagnosis of myocardial pumping efficiency.

The Swan Ganz Catheter is an important tool for use in the care of the critically ill patient, as it enables rapid treatment of potentially lethal cardiac dysfunction. It has been found that deterioration in the contractile performance of the left ventricle can be demonstrated during Swan Ganz monitoring before symptoms of heart failure present. As a result, treatment can commence before the appearance of such serious symptoms as pulmonary oedema. Before discussing Swan Ganz monitoring in detail, we should first revise the physiology of the normal heart.

De-oxygenated blood returns via the venous system to the right side of the heart. The right ventricle contracts and the blood is forced into the pulmonary artery, and thus into the lungs. The blood vessels within the lungs form a capillary network to reach each alveolus. Diffusion, and the exchange of oxygen and carbon dioxide, takes place across the alveolar and capillary membrane. Oxygenated blood then returns to the left side of the heart. The left atrium acts as reservoir for blood between contractions of the left ventricle. The blood

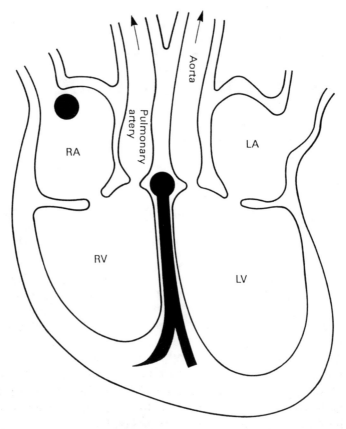

Figure 6.1 *Diagram of the heart.*

ejected from the left ventricle enters the arterial network of blood vessels through the aortic valve.

Cardiac output is not constant, for example it increases with exercise, but will decrease in response to diminished venous return or myocardial damage. Cardiac output is dependent on two factors: heart rate and stroke volume. The stroke volume is the amount of blood ejected from the ventricles at each contraction. Given an average heart rate of 72 beats per minute and a stroke volume of 70 ml per beat at rest, the cardiac output = 72 × 70 = approximately 5 litres per minute.

The stroke volume may increase to compensate for a slow rate. The increase in stroke volume occurs due to increased diastolic time which permits the ventricle a longer period for filling. If the heart rate becomes very slow then there are too few contractions to transfer blood from the venous to the arterial side, resulting in inadequate filling of the left ventricle and reduced cardiac output. However if the heart rate becomes very fast, diastolic filling time is shortened and inadequate filling may result.

In the healthy heart, the volume of blood available for pumping, the contractile strength of the myocardium and the degree of peripheral vascular resistance is finely balanced. In the diseased or compromised heart the fine balance mechanism is lost. The advantage of Swan Ganz monitoring is that it permits measurement of the heart's workload and its pumping ability. Three main factors govern cardiac efficiency and they may be described as follows.

1 Preload
Preload is the volume of blood in the ventricle at the end of diastole, i.e. the end diastolic volume. The pressure exerted on the walls, of the myocardium, can more easily be measured than the volume of the ventricle just prior to contraction. Left end diastolic pressure is therefore more likely to be used. This pressure is unfortunately altered should the left ventricular walls lose their elasticity, i.e. following anterior myocardial infarction. Venous return to the heart, venous tone, blood volume and the efficiency of the thoracic pump all affect the preload.

2 Contractile Inotropic State of the Myocardium
The ability of the myocardium to contract efficiently can be influenced by a number of factors:
- Myocardial infarction, in which the number of healthy contractile muscle fibres is reduced.
- The presence of sympathetic nerve activity and catecholamines, which are released as part of the stress response. This will increase myocardial contractility but may alter the stroke volume by shortening diastolic filling time.
- Hypoxia and acidosis effectively suppress myocardial contractility and efficiency.

3 Afterload
Contraction of the ventricle against the impedence of the arterial vessels is the third factor influencing stroke volume.

It will be seen that the greater the arterial resistance, the greater the force of contraction needs to be to overcome it. An example would be increased peripheral resistance due perhaps to hypothermia. The peripheral blood vessels shut down to conserve heat, causing a rise in preload and increasing the pressure in the arterial network. This increased load will cause alteration in the stroke volume and cardiac output.

Such changes in the pumping efficiency of the heart pose a serious threat to the patient. The Swan Ganz catheter gives a lot of useful information which can help to detect and treat potentially lethal changes in cardiac output.

PRESSURE MEASUREMENTS USING SWAN GANZ CATHETERS

The pressure within the right atrium is within the range of 0–8 mm Hg, varying with respirations. During diastole the pulmonary valve closes and the tricuspid valve opens, filling the right ventricle with blood. As the pressure rises in the right ventricle with filling, the tricuspid valve closes.

Contraction of the heart overcomes the pressure present in the pulmonary artery, causing the pulmonary valve to open and permitting the passage of blood. This is systole. During systole the right ventricular pressure is between 15–30 mm Hg, and during the diastole between 0–8 mm Hg.

The low pressure during diastole permits adequate filling from the atria, the higher pressure during systole permits ejection of blood into the pulmonary artery. The pressures within the pulmonary artery are 15–30 mm Hg during systole and 5–15 mm Hg during diastole.

The pulmonary capillaries also have a pressure gradient, and an open pathway leads from them via the pulmonary veins to the left ventricle. If the blood flow from the right side of the heart is occluded, the pressure exerted in the left side of the heart is transmitted back through the capillaries and can be measured, this is a good indicator of left sided heart function.

The pressure within the left atrium is between 4–12 mm Hg, in the left ventricle the pressure range is, 140–90 mm Hg during systole, and 4–12 mm Hg during diastole. As with the right side of the heart, these pressures are necessary to ensure adequate filling and ejection of blood.

Swan Ganz pressure monitoring utilizes these pressure gradients within the pulmonary circulation to monitor left heart function. Cannulation of the left atrium is potentially very hazardous for the patient, as dysrhythmias and trauma to the myocardium can seriously jeopardize cardiac output. Consequently indirect measurement via a Swan Ganz catheter is the usual method used to monitor left heart function.

There are three different types of catheters used:

1 **Double Lumen**

As with the other two types of Swan Ganz catheters, the double lumen has a small balloon approximately 1 mm from the tip of the catheter. One of the lumens is used to inflate the balloon with a preset amount of air, the other is used to take the measurements. When the balloon is in the right atrium it is inflated, and is able to float with the flow of blood into the right ventricle and pulmonary artery. As the catheter passes into the pulmonary arterial network it eventually reaches a vessel which is too small to allow it to pass any further, it will therefore wedge in this position. Blood flow from the right side of the heart cannot enter the vessel, and the pressure within the left side of the heart is transmitted back through the circulation to the catheter. With the catheter in this position, pulmonary venous pressure, left atrial pressure (LAP), and left ventricular end diastolic pressure (LVEDP) can be measured. The waveform can be displayed on a monitor at the patient's bedside.

This type of catheter can also be used to sample mixed venous blood in the pulmonary circulation and administer intravenous infusions.

2 **Triple Lumen**

This catheter has a third lumen which is at the proximal end of the catheter. When the catheter tip lies in the pulmonary artery the proximal lumen lies in the right atrium. This permits measurement of the right atrial pressure or central venous pressure (CVP). This lumen may also be used to give intravenous drugs and fluids.

3 **Thermodilution Catheter**

This catheter has three lumens and a thermistor at its distal end just proximal to the balloon (see Figure 6.2). The thermistor measures the temperature of blood flowing past the catheter. A small computer is needed when using the thermodilution catheter as the cardiac output is calculated by changes in temperature and flow. These computers are supplied by the manufacturers.

To measure the cardiac output an iced solution is injected through the proximal lumen which lies in the right atrium, the thermistor registers the change in blood temperature and the computer calculates the speed of blood flow and gives the cardiac output. Serial measurements are more valid than isolated readings due to the variable nature of cardiac output. It is common practice to take three measurements in succession.

INSERTION OF A SWAN GANZ CATHETER

Equipment

One Swan Ganz catheter, size 7 Fg for adult use, either double, treble, or thermodilution. If the catheter is not supplied with an insertion kit you will need:

- 1 introducer, size 8 Fg (the catheter threads through this as it is not rigid enough to cannulate a vein)
- 1 non return valve
- 1 extending sheath
- 1 scalpel
- 2 syringes, 10 ml x 1, 5 ml x 1
- Hypodermic needles size 21 g and 19 g
- Lignocaine 1% or 2%, 5 ml
- Gallipot and gauze swabs
- Chlorhexidine in spirit, skin preparation
- Suture material, usually 3/0 silk with a curved needle
- Needle holder
- Scissors
- Sterile towels x 2
- Gown
- Mask
- Surgeon gloves
- Dry iodine spray
- Sterile transparent occlusive dressing

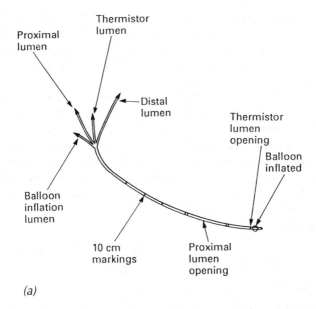

(a)

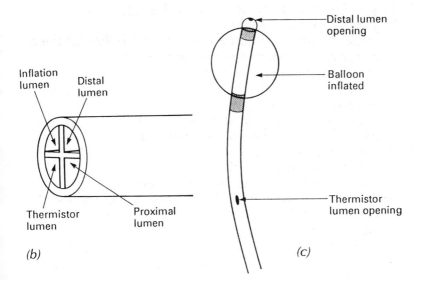

(b)   *(c)*

Figure 6.2   *(a) Swan Ganz catheter*
                    (b) Cross section of the Swan Ganz catheter
                    (c) Catheter tip in more detail.

The catheter balloon is inflated with a special graded syringe supplied with the catheter. Only this syringe should be used to inflate the balloon, as it is compatible with the catheter. It is luer locked and marked specifically to prevent over-inflation of the balloon.

Emergency resuscitation equipment and drugs should be available as insertion of the catheter through the heart may provoke dysrhythmias.

The commonest insertion site is the subclavian vein, although the ante-cubital fossa and femoral veins can also be used.

Preparation

A full explanation of the procedure is given to the patient. This may be a lengthy procedure and it is reassuring for the patient to have a nurse close by to explain what is happening. It may be necessary to cover part of the patient's face with a sterile towel to prevent contamination of the catheter. This may add to the patient's anxiety, especially if no explanation is given. Movement of the catheter through the heart may provoke a sensation of fluttering or pressure in the chest. The nurse can reassure the patient and monitor the response to this procedure. It is vital the patient remains still during insertion of the catheter, therefore the patient is made as comfortable as possible in bed in a supine position. Restrictive clothing is removed and the patient is kept warm. Dressings, jewellery and electrodes are removed from the insertion site.

Procedure (Subclavian Route)

The skin is cleaned and the sterile towels are positioned around the insertion site. The skin is infiltrated with local anaesthetic, which should be given sufficient time to work before, a small nick is made in the skin, this facilitates the passage of the introducer. The subclavian vein is cannulated and the non return valve attached to the end preventing the flow back of blood.

• The sterile extending sheath is attached to the valve, this maintains the sterility of the catheter and permits manipulation.

- The Swan Ganz catheter is flushed with saline, excluding all air bubbles, and the balloon is inflated to check patency.
- The catheter, with the balloon deflated, is passed through the sheath, valve and introducer, the pressure transducer set-up is attached to the distal lumen of the catheter.
- The Swan Ganz catheter is then advanced forwards until the pressure waveform on the monitor conforms to the usual right atrial waveform configuration (see Figure 6.3).
- The balloon is re-inflated and the catheter floats through the right ventricle into the pulmonary artery where it wedges in a pulmonary capillary, and the mean pressure is recorded (the pulmonary artery wedge pressure PAWP).
- In each part of the heart there will be a different pressure which may be identified as the catheter is passed through by the waveforms produced on the monitor.
- If the balloon is re-inflated, the catheter may be floated in the pulmonary artery, the systolic and diastolic pulmonary artery pressures (PAP) may then be displayed continuously on a monitor. Eventually the catheter will wedge in a branch of the pulmonary artery that is too narrow to permit its passage.
- This pressure is recorded as the pulmonary artery wedge pressure (PAWP). The proximal lumen can also be attached to a transducer and used for CVP measurements.
- Once correct positioning is obtained, the catheter insertion site is cleaned, sprayed with dry iodine spray and a transparent occlusive dressing applied. The patient is made comfortable in bed.
- Suturing of the introducer to the skin is dependent on hospital policy, and in some hospitals a chest X-ray is taken to confirm correct positioning and exclude pneumothorax.

MEASURING PULMONARY ARTERY WEDGE PRESSURE

This procedure is usually performed by medical staff. Nurses undertaking this procedure should have received specialist training and assessment under the auspices of the 'Extended Role' of the nurse policies in force in each health authority.

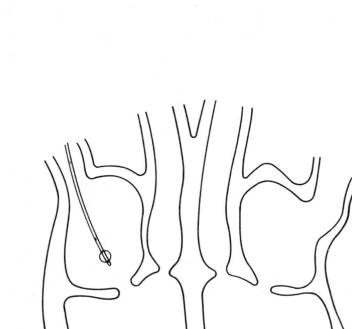

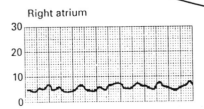

Right atrium

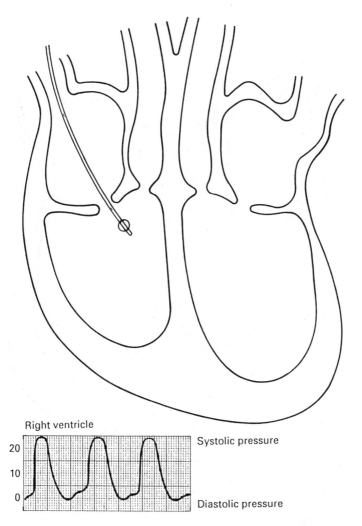

Right ventricle

20

10

0

Systolic pressure

Diastolic pressure

continued

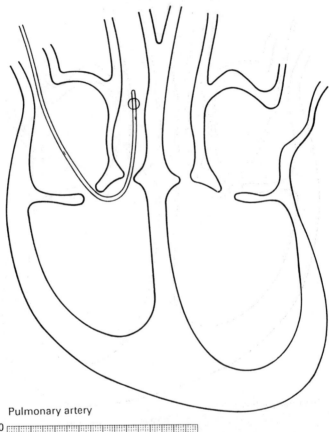

Pulmonary artery

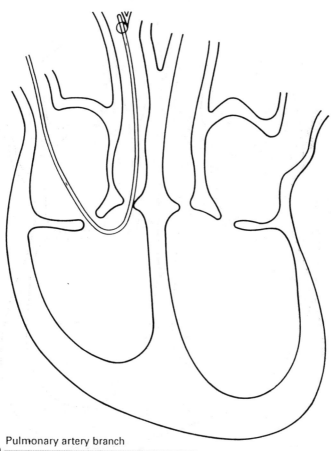

Pulmonary artery branch

continued

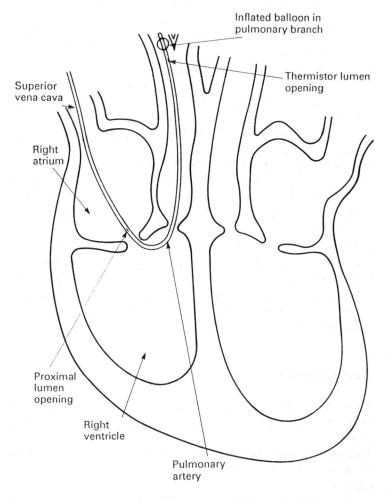

Figure 6.3 *Demonstrates the passage of the catheter through the heart and the waveforms produced.*

Procedure

1 Ensure the transducer is calibrated and level with the zero reference point.
2 Observe that the correct PAP waveform is displayed on the monitor.

3 Using the correct syringe, inflate the balloon using the recommended amount of air, some resistance to inflation will be felt in the syringe. Observe the monitor for changed waveform (see Figure 6.3).
4 Obtain and record the mean PAWP, the normal range being between 4–12 mm Hg. Levels higher than this may indicate left ventricular failure, mitral stenosis or insufficiency. However the PAWP may be kept at a higher level in the critically ill patient. Also take into account whether the patient is ventilated as this will affect the reading.
5 Gently deflate the balloon, most catheters have a two-way tap attached to the balloon lumen, this should be switched to the 'OFF' position to prevent accidental re-inflation of the balloon. Observe the monitor for restoration of the PAP waveform.
6 Ensure the alarm settings are in the 'ON' position.
7 Observe for dysrhythmia, and changes in the vital signs.
8 Remember that if the catheter balloon is left inflated, the section of lung distally will have had its blood supply cut off and will eventually infarct in the same way that would occur if the patient suffered a pulmonary embolism.

Troubleshooting

Apart from the problems related to transducer set-up and catheter misplacement a number of other problems may occur.
Problem: Pulmonary wedge waveform is not present when air has been injected into the balloon.
Causes
1 Incorrect amount of air in the balloon.
  Intervention: Deflate the balloon and inject the correct amount of air.
2 Balloon may be ruptured, this is noticeable if no resistance is felt when inflating the balloon.
  Intervention: Do not inject any more air. Obtain medical advice, remove catheter and replace if necessary.
3 Catheter not in the pulmonary artery.
  Intervention: Obtain medical advice. Remove catheter and replace if necessary. X-ray will confirm position of catheter.

Problem: Low, straight waveform on the monitor.
Causes
1 Catheter may be occluded with blood.
    Intervention: Do not irrigate, but attempt gentle aspirations through the distal lumen. Obtain medical advice, remove and replace catheter if necessary.
2 Catheter tip occluded by vessel wall.
    Intervention: Deflate the balloon. Consult a doctor, who can if necessary withdraw the catheter 1–2 cm.
3 Transducer is not securely attached to the catheter.
    Intervention: Check security of all connections in the pressure set up.

Problem: Pressure waveform changes suddenly.
Causes:
1 Air or blood in the equipment.
    Intervention: Check the security of all the connections and evacuate all air or blood.
2 Transducer not calibrated.
    Intervention: Recalibrate the transducer and check level against the zero reference point.

Nursing Management of the Patient Undergoing Swan Ganz Monitoring

Nursing management of a patient with Swan Ganz monitoring is similar to that of arterial monitoring. Close observation of the patient and equipment is vital in both cases. The reader is referred to Chapter 5 for monitoring information, transducer care and troubleshooting.

Precautions

1 Ensure that the alarms are set at all times. The settings should be 15–20 mm Hg above and below the patients pressure readings.
2 Ensure luer connections are secure.
3 Ensure equipment is free from air bubbles.
4 It is good practice to have a reference diagram of each waveform close at hand to assist with identification. Frequent checking to ensure the catheter remains in the

pulmonary artery is important because of the high risk of dysrhythmias if it floats back into the right ventricle.

5 Ensure medical staff are alerted promptly to changes in the pressure waveforms and readings.

6 Ensure the balloon is fully deflated following each measurement of wedge pressure, because occlusion of pulmonary vessels for prolonged periods may result in infarction of lung tissue.

7 Ensure the catheter is removed within 48 hours of insertion.

Potential Complications Associated with Swan Ganz Monitoring

- Air embolus
- Thromboembolism
- Pneumo/haemothorax
- Dysrhythmias
- Infection
- Cardiac tamponade
- Balloon rupture
- Lung ischaemia
- Pulmonary artery rupture
- Haemorrhage
- Pulmonary infarction

Catheter Removal

This precedure should be performed by medical staff with nursing assistance, although in some hospitals, nurses may remove Swan Ganz catheters under the auspices of the extended role of the nurse.

Action (1): Obtain baseline readings of blood pressure, heart rate and respiratory rate.
Rationale: To detect any changes from the baseline.

Action (2): Ensure ECG monitoring is in progress.
Rationale: Risk of dysrhythmias, increases as the catheter is withdrawn through the right ventricle, especially VT.

Action (3): Ensure the balloon is fully deflated.
Rationale: To permit withdrawal.

Action (4): With gloved hands gently retract the catheter.
Rationale: Rapid removal may provoke dysrhythmias or cause trauma to the myocardium. Gloves help to prevent cross infection by blood borne bacteria.

Action (5): Remove catheter fully and discard extending sheath.
Rationale: Swan Ganz catheters are for single use only.

Action (6): If appropriate remove the introducer.

Action (7): Apply firm pressure dressing over the wound site.
Rationale: If the femoral or ante-cubital fossa routes are used, firm pressure must be applied over the site for 10 minutes or, until the bleeding stops, to prevent haematoma formation.

Action (8): Spray the insertion site with dry iodine spray and apply a sterile transparent occlusive dressing.
Rationale: To prevent infection.

Action (9): Check wound insertion site frequently.
Rationale: Observe for haemorrhage for up to six hours following removal of catheter.

Action (10): Ensure the Swan Ganz catheter is intact.
Rationale: Inflate the balloon to ensure it is present eliminating the risk of leaving parts of the catheter within the patient's body.

Action (11): Record vital signs at least hourly for the first six hours following removal of catheter.
Rationale: Observe for signs of reactive haemorrhage and shock.

The following medical conditions require the use of Swan Ganz techniques in the critically ill patient.

Acute Pulmonary Oedema

In this condition, the left ventricle does not fully empty at systole and therefore becomes over distended increasing pre-load. Filling of the ventricle from the atria increases the distention of the ventricle and so increases the pre-load. For a while the increased pre-load helps to maintain the cardiac output, but usually the pre-load continues to rise causing loss of myocardial contractility due to over-stretching of the myocardial fibres. The cardiac output falls, as does the stroke volume and progressively, the amount of blood remaining in the ventricles increases. The left atrium dilates, as it cannot fully empty prior to systole. This in turn causes a back pressure of blood in the pulmonary veins and capillaries. The pressure of this blood causes fluid from the circulation to enter the interstitial spaces and the alveoli, in the lung. This is pulmonary oedema.

Pulmonary oedema increases the distance oxygen molecules have to travel across the alveolar membrane to reach the blood. As a result, arterial oxygen levels fall. Within the alveolus, oedema reduces the surface area available for oxygen and carbon dioxide gaseous exchange, leading to hypoxia and hypercapnia. The symptoms include, dyspnoea, sweating and anxiety. The clinical signs include, cyanosis, haemoptysis (pink frothy sputum), the presence of rhonchi and basal crepitations in the chest, and diffuse shadowing of the lung field on X-ray.

Cardiogenic Shock

This is usually defined as shock caused directly by myocardial damage. More commonly it occurs following myocardial infarction, usually an anterior infarction, although rupture of the ventricular septum and acute mitral regurgitation may also be causes. The clinical signs include hypotension, with a systolic blood pressure below 90 mm Hg, urine output falls to below 20 ml/hour, impaired mental function and peripheral vasoconstriction resulting in cold, clammy skin. Pulmonary oedema may be a further symptom. Increased preload and afterload associated with reduced myocardial contractility may present during cardiogenic shock.

Chronic Left Heart Failure

Hypertrophy, or enlargement of the heart may occur as a coping mechanism when a chronic increase in pressure is imposed on the heart. Each of the myocardial fibres increases in size attempting to improve contractile strength, progressively this leads to gross enlargement of the heart.

Signs develop more slowly and include dyspnoea, orthopnoea (the necessity for an upright posture for adequate breathing) and paroxysmal nocturnal dyspnoea. Chronic preload and afterload stresses are associated with left heart failure.

Right Heart Failure

Hypertrophy of the right ventricle (due to its inability to cope with the demands made on it), and tricuspid stenosis lead to right heart failure. Right heart failure may also follow as a consequence of left ventricular failure (congestive cardiac failure), pulmonary disease, and pulmonary and tricuspid diseases. Symptoms of pulmonary disease, cor pulmonale, may be present. These include dyspnoea, pain and haemoptysis. Raised venous pressure due to right heart failure causes enlargement of the liver, which may become cirrhotic, and gravity dependent oedema of the legs, and occasionally ascites.

Major Trauma

Swan Ganz monitoring can also be a useful tool in the diagnosis and treatment of complications due to massive blood transfusion in the multiply injured. ARDS (Adult Respiratory Distress Syndrome) and multi-organ failure often occur following massive blood transfusion and may be related to the storage time of the blood, although ARDS may also occur in any number of other conditions unrelated to blood transfusion. The symptoms of ARDS include dyspnoea, tachypnoea and cyanosis developing over a period of 12 to 48 hours after injury. The patient has severe hypoxaemia and lung compliance falls. Chest X-ray reveals widespread opacification. The management of the patient includes careful administration of fluids, and optimizing oxygen transport and cardiac output.

Septicaemic Shock

Septic shock is unlike the other forms of shock described in previous chapters in that instead of reducing cardiac output, and therefore tissue perfusion, the patient may well have a normal or increased cardiac output. The tissues may have access to oxygen and nutrients but are unable to use them effectively. Septic shock may be caused by bacteria or their toxic products and as a result blood cultures may be negative. The symptoms of septic shock are varied; in the early stages the patient may be febrile, tachypnoeic and vaso dilated. The patient may have a hyperdynamic circulation and urine output may be reduced or increased. If symptoms of septicaemic shock are not recognized and treated, the more usual symptoms of shock with hypotension and peripheral vasoconstriction may then occur. Monitoring of the patient using a Swan Ganz catheter permits early detection of this condition. Therapy may include manipulation of the patients preload and afterload. The contractility of the myocardium can also be supported and improved using drugs like Dobutamine. Maintenance of cardiac output is of paramount importance as it may be a major determinant of the patient's survival.

Pulmonary Emboli

The Swan Ganz catheter can also be used to administer streptokinase by infusion directly into the pulmonary circulation to dissolve clots. In certain circumstances emboli form in the pulmonary circulation and cause infarction of lung tissue. Massive embolization within the pulmonary circulation gives rise to symptoms of shock. The patient may complain of a pleuritic type of chest pain. The effects of embolization on the circulation are increased pulmonary artery pressure, due to mechanical obstruction, hypoxia, and decreased cardiac output. Cardiopulmonary resuscitation and treatment for shock may be necessary. Streptokinase is a plasminogen activator and is given in severe cases within 48 hours of acute onset. Streptokinase causes lysis of the clot but has two main disadvantages: bleeding and allergic reactions.

Recent surgery, uncontrolled hypertension, peptic ulceration and recent trauma are all contraindicates for the use of streptokinase. Heparin by infusion is also usually given in conjunction with streptokinase. When thrombolytic therapy is used it is vital that emergency drugs are readily available and the patient must be closely monitored. If complications occur, fresh frozen plasma can be given to counteract the effects of the streptokinase. Epsilon aminocaproic acid can also be used to rapidly antagonize streptokinase. The advantages to the patient of Swan Ganz and CVP monitoring can, despite the risks, be very great. A critically ill patient is always at risk of circulatory overload and consequently pulmonary oedema and heart failure. The accurate information that is available as a result of these techniques greatly assist the medical staff in trying to avoid serious complications.

SWAN GANZ MONITORING — EXERCISES

1 List the causes of heart failure.
2 Describe the symptoms of acute pulmonary oedema.
3 What do you understand by the term wedge pressure?
4 List the complications of Swan Ganz catheterization that the nurse should be looking for.
5 What are the normal pressure ranges within the left and right ventricles?

7

Intracranial Pressure Monitoring

Intracranial pressure monitoring is a useful procedure of evaluating cerebral pathology. In the general intensive therapy unit (ITU), intracranial pressure (ICP) monitoring is used to observe and assess the effects of raised intracranial pressure on the severely head injured patient. ICP monitoring also gives important information relating to cerebral function, and therefore permits prompt and accurate treatment of raised ICP. The procedure has many other applications, as it may be used in the assessment and treatment of conditions which can be classified as intracerebral or systemic.

Intracerebral conditions including head injury, tumours, sub-arachnoid haemorrhage, intracranial haemorrhage, hydrocephalus, cerebral ischaemia and infection including meningitis. Intracranial monitoring is mainly used for observation of intracerebral conditions. Systemic conditions include hypertension causing vascular thrombosis, metabolic encephalitis, infection, sceptacaemia, hypoxia and hypercarbia.

The brain and spinal cord are encased in bone. The skull and vertebrae being the main defence against potential injury. The brain and spinal cord are covered by three separate tissue layers, the meninges. These structures are:

- Dura mater, this is a thick fibrous outer membrane, which is adherent to the underside of the skull.
- The arachnoid mater, a vascular membrane involved in the production and reabsorbtion of cerebro spinal fluid, (CSF). A potential space exists between the dura and arachoid membranes.
- The pia mater, a fine membrane which lies in very close

proximity to the brain tissue. A space exists between the arachnoid and pia maters, which contains cerebro spinal fluid. This is the subarachnoid space.

CEREBROSPINAL FLUID

CSF is a clear, electrolyte solution, which circulates round the brain tissue, via the cerebral ventricles and subarachnoid space. CSF maintains uniform pressure around the cerebral structures, acting as a water bath, the brain remaining buoyant in this solution. CSF contains electrolytes and glucose. A limited amount of low molecular weight protein is also present within CSF.

CSF is manufactured by the choroid plexus in the ventricles of the brain, and in certain of the cerebral blood vessels. CSF closely matches, in its composition, the extracellular fluid surrounding the neurones.

The cerebral ventricles, of which there are four are connected to each other to permit the flow of CSF between them. It also circulates around the brain and spinal cord in the subarachnoid space. The CSF is then reabsorbed by the arachnoid villi, and is recirculated or removed through the venous sinuses. Reabsorbtion of CSF, by the arachnoid vessels for recirculation, is suppressed if the ICP rises above certain limits. Production of CSF is not however influenced by raised intraventricular pressure. A blockage present within the CSF circulatory pathway can therefore lead to hydrocephalus, as despite the blockage, CSF will continue to be produced. The normal amount of CSF present within the brain and spinal cord is approximately 125 ml, and the total flow per day, through the brain tissue is approximately 500 ml.

CEREBRAL BLOOD CIRCULATION

The blood vessels supplying the brain, are the internal carotids, the vertebral arteries and the anterior spinal artery. The vertebral arteries combine to form the basilar artery, this with the internal carotids forms the circle of Willis. The anterior spinal artery contributes to the blood supply of the medulla.

The circle of Willis forms an uninterrupted pathway for arterial blood to the brain tissue. The circle formation protects the brain tissue from ischaemia, because should one of the vessels lose its patency there will always be an alternative route available, (see Figure 7.1).

The capillaries, within the brain, are very similar to those found in other parts of the body but they are however different, as they have a tendency to be selectively permeable. This selective permeability results in the blood brain barrier through which water, carbon dioxide and oxygen can pass readily, however glucose takes longer and electrolytes even longer still. The function of the barrier is probably to maintain a constant environment around the neurones, and minimize any changes that might occur. Many drugs cannot cross this barrier, which limits the range of drug therapies available for treatment of cerebral disease. This explains the use of sulphonamides and penicillin, in the treatment of intracerebral infections, as they are the most effective antibiotics at crossing the blood brain barrier. The venous drainage from the brain is via deep veins and large sinuses in the dura, which empty into the internal jugular veins.

Cerebral Blood Flow

Due to the encasement of the brain, within rigid bone, any increase in fluid within the brain cannot readily be compensated for by an expansion in cerebral volume. Once swelling of brain tissue occurs, or if there is haemorrhage or a tumour present, pressure increases must occur. This leads to a reduction in cerebral blood flow and venous drainage from the brain. This in turn causes oedema and ischaemia. Interruption in the formation, flow, and excretion of CSF compounds this problem.

Reduction in cerebral blood flow may provoke changes in pH, carbon dioxide (pCO_2) and oxygen (pO_2) tensions in arterial blood. Hypercarbia and hypoxia produce vasodilation of intracerebral blood vessels, which combine to further increase ICP. This vicious circle can lead to herniation of brain

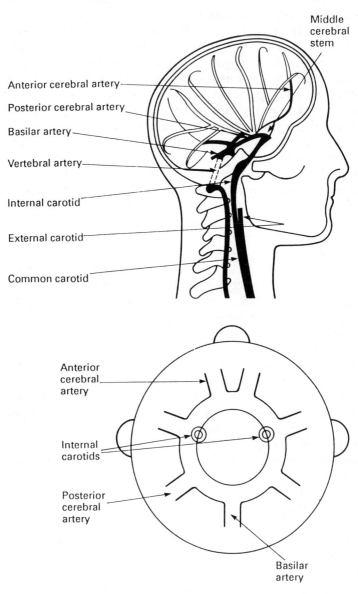

Figure 7.1   *Circle of Willis.*

tissue, through the foramen magnum, distorting the brain and causing mid-line shift. Herniation of brain tissue is often fatal.

Raised ICP even for a short period may reduce cerebral blood flow leading to ischaemia. In this situation the vasomotor centre is stimulated, causing a rise in systemic blood pressure in an attempt to increase cerebral blood flow. The cardiorespiratory centres are also stimulated causing bradycardia and reduced respiratory rate. (The opposite reflex to shock and a falling blood pressure). A further complicating factor in this series of events is the redistribution of blood to parts of the brain, initially unaffected by the raised pressure. These areas effectively 'steal' vital oxygenated blood from the damaged part of the brain, increasing its hypoxia and ischaemic damage. The increase in blood pressure however causes a general increase in pressure within the brain, leading to global oedema.

SYMPTOMS OF RAISED INTRACRANIAL PRESSURE

These symptoms are dependent on the degree of injury and the speed of onset and increase of pressure. Headache, vomiting and papilloedema may present in the early stages, along with a variable decrease in response to Glasgow coma scale testing. Symptoms associated with ischaemia include, fixed dilated pupils, hypertension, unconsciousness, apnoea and suppression of brain stem reflexes. Distortion of the brain tissue produces symptoms of, drowsiness, headache and vomiting. Decerebrate rigidity, pupillary changes, bradycardia, hypertension, respiratory abnormalities and altered brain stem reflexes may also be present. It should be remembered however, that just as no two people are completely alike, the range of presenting symptoms will also be very variable.

Treatment of Raised Intracranial Pressure

In most general ITU wards the patient's admitted with raised ICP are the victims of trauma. It is beyond the remit of this book to discuss the varied and specific treatments given for cerebral injuries or diseases, and therefore a general approach to the subject will be taken.

On admission to hospital and thereafter it is important to assess the extent of cerebral dysfunction. In the initial stages this includes observation, examination and assessment of levels of consciousness and response to stimuli. In Britain the standard methods of assessment of cerebral function are as set out by the Glasgow coma scale (see Figure 7.2).

GLASGOW COMA SCALE

As can be seen in Figure 7.2, this scale permits assessment of the level of consciousness and response to stimuli by a number of standardized tests including:

Eye Opening: Either spontaneously, to speech or to painful stimuli. This indicates depth of coma and arousal, but does not reflect patient awareness or orientation.

Verbal Response: These responses are graded as orientated, confused, inappropriate, incomprehensible or none.

- **Orientated:** The patient converses cogently and lucidly and demonstrates awareness of time and place.
- **Confused:** The patient converses inappropriately and may appear disorientated to time and place.
- **Inappropriate:** This may be rambling speech, sometimes shouting but not in response to conversation.
- **Incomprehensible:** This presents as moaning and unintelligible words and sounds.

The presence of an endotracheal tube will obviously prevent the testing of these responses.

Best Motor Response: Where the patient is unable to obey commands, a painful stimulus is used to elicit responses. The recommended method of delivering a painful stimuli is nail bed pressure with a pen. This prevents over enthusiastic testing by pinching or twisting the ear lobes, or rubbing the sternum with the knuckles. These methods serve only to cause bruising of the skin and worry to the relatives.

The best motor response is a normal movement of a limb in response to a painful stimuli, i.e. flexion or withdrawal from pain. The response will vary with the degree of cerebral damage:

1 Localized, the patient withdraws the limb being tested.

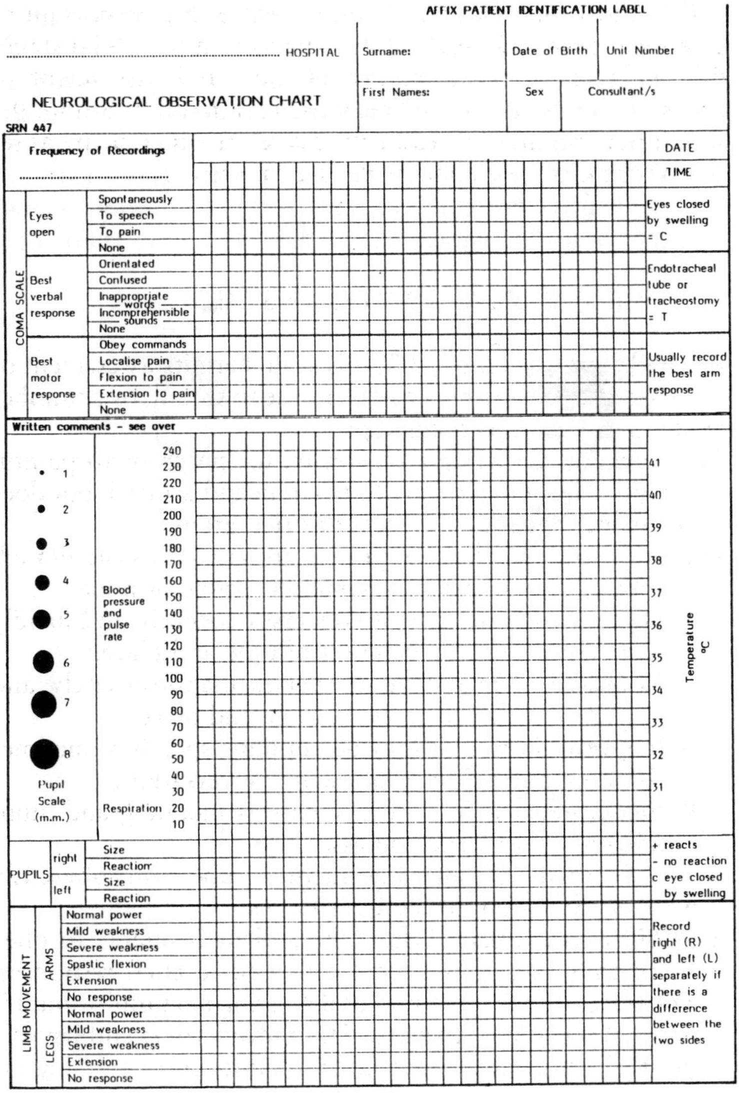

AFFIX PATIENT IDENTIFICATION LABEL

.... HOSPITAL

Surname:	Date of Birth	Unit Number
First Names:	Sex	Consultant/s

NEUROLOGICAL OBSERVATION CHART

SRN 447

Frequency of Recordings .... | DATE | TIME

COMA SCALE

- Eyes open: Spontaneously; To speech; To pain; None — Eyes closed by swelling = C
- Best verbal response: Orientated; Confused; Inappropriate words; Incomprehensible sounds; None — Endotracheal tube or tracheostomy = T
- Best motor response: Obey commands; Localise pain; Flexion to pain; Extension to pain; None — Usually record the best arm response

Written comments – see over

Pupil Scale (m.m.): 1, 2, 3, 4, 5, 6, 7, 8

Blood pressure and pulse rate: 240, 230, 220, 210, 200, 190, 180, 170, 160, 150, 140, 130, 120, 110, 100, 90, 80, 70, 60, 50, 40, 30, 20, 10

Respiration

Temperature °C: 41, 40, 39, 38, 37, 36, 35, 34, 33, 32, 31

PUPILS: right – Size, Reaction; left – Size, Reaction — + reacts; - no reaction; c eye closed by swelling

LIMB MOVEMENT

- ARMS: Normal power; Mild weakness; Severe weakness; Spastic flexion; Extension; No response
- LEGS: Normal power; Mild weakness; Severe weakness; Extension; No response

Record right (R) and left (L) separately if there is a difference between the two sides

Figure 7.2 *A neurological observation chart.*

2 Flexor movement of one or more limbs.
3 Extensor movement. This abnormal response is taken to indicate that the patient is decerebrate, it may manifest itself in two ways:

- Decerebrate rigidity, (Figure 7.3), in response to stimuli the patient adopts a rigid posture with extension of all limbs and arching of the back. The patient may hyperventilate, and the limbs appear to quiver with the effort of remaining stretched.
- Decorticate rigidity, (Figure 7.3), in response to stimuli the hands clench and the arms are held in flexion against the chest. The patient's legs adopt the extensor posture.

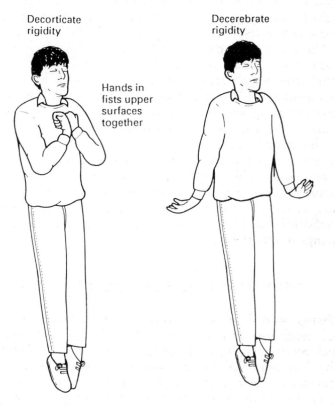

Decorticate rigidity

Decerebrate rigidity

Hands in fists upper surfaces together

Figure 7.3 *Diagram of postures adopted by patients following head injury.*

Both of these postures demonstrate significant intracerebral dysfunction.

In some cases no response will be elicited and the limbs are flaccid. Apart from catastrophic cerebral disorders, this state may be induced by drugs, i.e. muscle relaxants like pancuronium. The size of the pupil is controlled by the third cranial nerve, (occulmotor). This nerve runs over the surface of the brain and in the presence of localized swelling (e.g. haematoma) may be compressed. The result is a decrease in nerve function, relaxation of muscle and dilation of the pupil. Assessment of pupil size is therefore an important factor. The coma scale gives a comparison set of pupil sizes in millimetres for use at the bedside. Following this assessment a bright light is shone into each eye in turn and the pupil observed for size and speed of response, i.e. sluggish, rapid, dilated fixed etc.

The coma scale gives objective and reliable information about the patient's cerebral status. The recordings form a trend from which valuable information can be elicited, and treatment given for deteriorating cerebral function. In the initial stages quarter hourly observations are vital as haemorrhage and oedema may occur rapidly.

The strength of the Glasgow coma scale is that two different observers may use it on the same patient and end up with the same results. This is unlikely if such terms as 'drowsy' or 'semiconscious' were used to describe level of consciousness. Any change in the level of consciousness can therefore confidently said to be real changes rather than reflecting a change in observer.

INTRACRANIAL PRESSURE (ICP) MONITORING

Changes in ICP can occur suddenly following head injury and ICP monitoring gives an immediate and continuous record of such pressure changes. The use of Computer Axial Tomography Scanning (CAT) techniques of the head can reveal the presence of haemorrhage, oedema and shifts or distortion of brain tissue following trauma. The CAT scan has the disadvantage of being a single picture at one point in time, compared to the continuous information obtained from ICP monitoring. This information can be used to decide and evaluate the treatment used for raised intracranial pressure.

The ICP, measured in a patient resting quietly in the supine position, is approximately 10 mm Hg (1.3 kPa). This pressure is related to the production and reabsorption of cerebrospinal fluid and cerebral blood volume. In all cases increase in one component relating to the maintenance of a uniform intracranial pressure, (e.g. CSF production) must cause a decrease in another, (e.g. CSF reabsorption). The intracranial volume is fixed, although there is some 'give' in the system. The intracranial contents are composed of:

- Brain and intracellular water   80–85%
- Cerebro spinal fluid   5–12%
- Cerebral blood flow   3– 7%

Although the cerebral blood volume makes up the smallest percentage of intracranial contents, it responds rapidly to changes in pressure within the brain. The intracranial pressure will only remain normal as long as the compensation mechanisms within the brain can cope.

Cerebral perfusion pressure (CPP) is the difference between the mean cerebral arterial pressure and the mean cerebral venous pressure. The cerebral perfusion pressure is the amount of pressure required to perfuse all of the brain tissue, this of course varies in the presence of injury and ischaemia. In the supine patient the cerebral arterial pressure is equal to the systemic blood pressure. Cerebral perfusion pressure is most easily calculated by subtracting the intracranial pressure from the mean arterial pressure. This is important to consider as in the head injured patient, hypertension is a common symptom, and attemps made to reduce systemic blood pressure will compromise the cerebral perfusion pressure. For example, in the head injured patient, if the mean arterial pressure is 100 mm Hg (13.3 kPa) and the ICP is 40 mm Hg (5.3 kPa), the cerebral perfusion pressure is 60 mm Hg (8.0 kPa) which is the level of pressure required to perfuse the brain. By reducing the mean arterial pressure the cerebral perfusion pressure is also reduced potentiating further ischaemia.

Using intraventricular or subdural monitoring it will be seen that the pressure waveform is dynamic and pulsatile. This is due to cerebral blood vessel pulsation, the degree of cerebral tissue compliance, the patient's position in bed and the effects of respiration. The 'normal' level of ICP is approximately 10 mm Hg (1.3 kPa), but intracranial hypertension and associated symptoms which require treatment, may create a wide variety of pressure readings. The level of pressure at which treatment is initiated is not clearly defined. Some patients with ICP readings of 15 mm Hg (2.0 kPa) may have symptoms of raised intracranial pressure, i.e. decorticate or decerebrate signs, which must be treated, others may not have symptoms until a mean pressure of 25 mm Hg (3.3 kPa) or greater is reached. The patient must therefore be carefully observed and symptoms reported promptly to permit early intervention especially unusual changes in ICP readings lasting for longer than five minutes.

Although there are three distinct pressure waves visible on the ICP trace only the 'A' waves are the most significant (see Figure 7.4). 'B' and 'C' waves which may be present are not particularly helpful in assessing and evaluating the patient's treatment. 'A' waves are large increases of approximately 50 mm Hg (6.6 kPa) or greater above an established baseline of 20 mm Hg (2.7 kPa). These waves are associated with neurological symptoms and directly relate to rises in ICP. As a result the presence of 'A' waves indicates the necessity of prompt treatment. If the ICP continues to increase the baseline reading will also rise, and the 'A' waves will increase in size, duration and frequency. These waves are associated with increased cerebral blood volume and decreased cerebral blood flow.

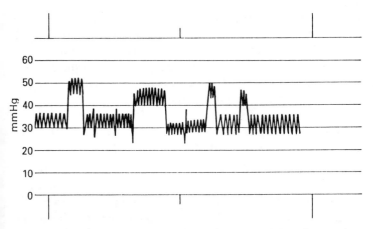

Figure 7.4   *'A' Waves (plateau waves) associated with raised intracranial pressure.*

Several methods of ICP monitoring are available using either, an epidural sensor, an intraventricular cannula or a subdural screw device. Each system has its advocates and except for the subdural monitoring method they are accurate indicators of cerebral pressure. The use of these techniques is dependent on the facilities available in the unit and hospital.

EPIDURAL ICP MONITORING

The sensor device, (see Figure 7.5), is 10 mm x 1 mm and is attached by cable to a monitor. The sensor is an air filled balloon containing a mirror, which moves in response to changes in ICP. Fibre optic threads transmit light between sensor and monitor. When no pressure is exerted on the balloon, the mirror is in close proximity to the fibre optic threads and light bounces off the mirror and returns along the cable to the monitor, where it is recorded. An increase in ICP causes the position of the mirror to change and therefore the direction of reflected light, back to the monitor is also changed. Bellows within the sensor balloon adjusts the pressure to equal ICP in the balloon. This returns the mirror to its normal position, opposite the fibre-optic threads. The pressure at the bellows is measured by an electrical transducer and it is displayed as a number on the monitor.

The device is inserted by a neuro surgeon, in the operating theatre under a general anaesthetic, through a small burr hole in the skull. The dura is stripped away from the bone as the sensor will lie between bone and dura. The skin is sutured and a light dressing applied. The cable is attached to the monitor and continuous readings may then be taken.

Nursing Role

This procedure requires minimal nursing input, although frequent observation of the patient's neurological and cardiovascular status are vital. Although the monitor records pressure changes within the skull, the procedure is not infallible. The equipment, although generally reliable, may malfunction, and it is important that any deterioration in the patient's

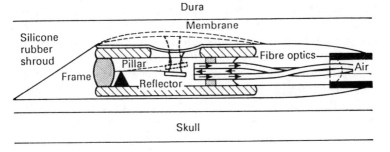

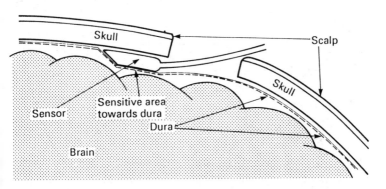

Figure 7.5   *(a) Epidural sensor device*
*(b) Positioning of epidural sensor device within
the skull.*

neurological state is reported rapidly to ensure prompt treatment. The measurement attained by this technique must be
interpreted in conjuction with the cardiovascular and neurological observations, recorded by the nurse, and not in
isolation.

The nurse should document transient rises in the ICP, these
changes are often due to the patient experiencing pain or
coughing, both of which must be treated quickly to prevent
exacerbation of cerebral irritation. Rises in the ICP which
cannot be attributed to pain or coughing and are not transient
should be reported promptly. If the rise in ICP is thought to be
due to increased cerebral oedema, rather than haemorrhage,

the first line of treatment may be administration of a measured dose of mannitol 20%. Mannitol is an osmotic diuretic, the effect of which is to reduce blood volume and intracranial pressure. If however the raised ICP does not respond to drugs or if haemorrhage is suspected, or a lesion which is operable then burr holes, craniotomy or CAT scan may be considered.

Another important intervention would be careful monitoring of fluid balance. As the brain is already under considerable stress, overloading the circulation with fluid may further raise the ICP. It is usual to restrict fluids to approximately two litres per day, this is sufficient for the patient's needs but does not overfill the circulation. Careful administration of intravenous fluids must also be a priority, accidental over-administration of intravenous fluids will significantly contribute to an already raised ICP.

The incidence of intracerebral infection, following this procedure is reported as low, however the nurse must carefully observe the patient for signs of meningism. The insertion site must also be checked for signs of infection, and the wound must be dressed using an aseptic technique. As with all head injured patients, the bed head must remain higher than the foot as the head down position promotes raised intracranial pressure.

The monitor is calibrated prior to insertion of the sensor device, and does not need further calibration. The monitor cable can be disconnected, for movement of the patient and then reinserted on return. Pressure alarm settings can be set, to warn of changes in the ICP outside fixed limits.

Removal of the device is performed by medical staff. The sutures need to be removed, before it can be withdrawn. The skin is then resutured and dressed.

The sensor devices are very delicate and cannot withstand the usual sterilizing methods available in hospitals. The recommended method of sterilization is by ethylene oxide. This method is available in two or three centres in England, which means that after use, the device is sent to one of these centres for sterilizing. This process may in some cases take up to six weeks and is expensive.

Compared with other methods, this technique has the disadvantage of not permitting access for drainage or sampling of CSF.

INTRAVENTRICULAR METHOD

This technique involves insertion of a catheter into the anterior ventricle via a burr hole (see Figure 7.6). It is connected via a three-way tap and tubing to a transducer dome and monitor. The tubing and catheter are primed with sterile saline solution. The catheter is inserted in theatre under a general anaesthetic.

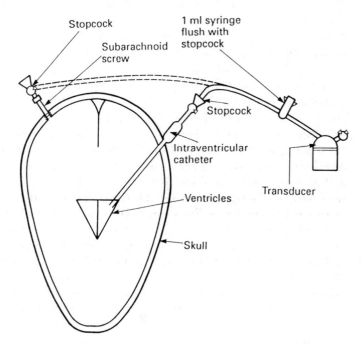

Figure 7.6   *Intracranial pressure monitoring using subarachnoid and intraventricular methods.*

Set-up for Intraventricular Monitoring

Equipment

- 1 transducer dome
- 3 x three-way taps.
- Sterile saline solution (0.9%) for priming

See Figure 7.6 for diagram of set procedure.

Action

1 Fill the transducer dome, pressure tubing and three-way taps with sterile priming solution.
2 Ensure air bubbles are evacuated.
   Rationale: Air bubbles pose a potential risk to the patient of embolization and they also damp the monitor trace.
3 Ensure all connections are secure.
   Rationale: Prevents leakage of cerebro spinal fluid from the patient.
4 Position transducer at level of the lateral ventricles.
   Rationale: This maintains accurate readings and prevents drainage of CSF when the set-up is attached to the patient.
5 Calibrate and zero the transducer, by venting to atmosphere and adjusting the calibration settings. Ensure sterility of the set-up maintained.
6 Medical staff will attach set-up to ventricular cannula.
7 Turn set-up 'ON' to patient and monitor by correct positioning of the three-way taps.
8 Check the waveform is sharply defined.
   Rationale: Damping of the trace may be due to misplacement of the catheter. Misaligned transducer or air bubbles in the set-up.
9 Ensure that the head of the bed remains at the level ordered and ensure that the transducers remain at the level of the ventricles.
10 Never reconnect tubing which has become disconnected, turn off three-way taps and seek medical assistance.

Nursing Role

The same interventions must be observed as for epidural ICP monitoring. This procedure however does involve more potential risks to the patient. The risk of infection can be high. Infection within the cerebral ventricles will have catastrophic effects on the patient. The nurse must make every effort to prevent the risks of infection by ensuring strict aseptic technique is used whilst manipulating the set-up or dressing the head wound.

A further hazard of the procedure is accidental drainage of CSF. This may occur due to loose connections in the tubing or patient manipulation. It is the nurses responsibility to ensure that all the connections are secure and patent, and that the patient is never left unattended. Air embolization may also occur if air bubbles are present within the tubing set-up, careful observation will help prevent this occurring.

This method of intrancranial monitoring permits sampling of the CSF for chemical analysis. Drainage of excessive amounts of CSF can also be performed. The disadvantage of the technique include increased risk of infection, and difficulty in locating ventricles in patients who have brain distortion, mid-line shift or small ventricles.

SUBARACHNOID PRESSURE MONITORING

See Figure 7.6 for diagram of set-up which closely resembles that of intraventricular monitoring. This method requires insertion of a hollow screw like device through a burr hole in the skull. The dura is opened and the device is placed 1 mm approximately below the level of the dura, in the subarachnoid space. The device is connected via a fluid filled set-up to a transducer and monitor. This method is largely being abandoned in many hospitals as it is unreliable and often inaccurate. The risk of infection is also high. Nursing care is as for intraventricular monitoring.

Treatment of Raised Intracranial Pressure

Once accurate recording of increased intracranial pressure is possible treatment can be closely evaluated and tailored to suit the patient's needs. The treatment of raised intracranial pressure includes:

1 **Fluid Restriction**: The patient is restricted to two litres per day. This prevents overloading of the circulation and assists the lowering of the intracranial pressure.
2 **Hyperventilation**: Prevention of hypoxia, and hypercarbia reduces cerebral oedema, dilation of cerebral blood vessels and consequently ischaemia.
3 **Drugs**: The use of anaesthetic drugs, i.e. thiopentone by continuous infusion, prevents restlessness and reduces tissue oxygen demand and heat production from muscle

movement. The use of mannitol, a hyperosmotic agent, causes a diuresis and helps to reduce ICP by removing cerebral and systemic water.

Aspirin and Paracetamol may also be prescribed for their anti-pyretic action. Heat is a potent vasodilator both in the skin and in the cerebral blood vessels.

4 Drainage of CSF may be carried out if an intraventricular cannula is in situ. Manual drainage of fluid will reduce ICP.

5 Craniotomy and removal of a bone flap in selected cases may decompress the brain tissue. Head injured patients provide a challenge for medical and nursing services. Prompt effective treatment of raised intracranial pressure influences the prognosis and the degree of rehabilitation possible. Close observation and prompt reporting of changes in the patient's clinical state are imperative if the patient is to regain a normal quality of life.

INTRACRANIAL PRESSURE MONITORING — EXERCISES

1 What do you understand by the blood brain barrier?
2 How does this barrier affect the drug therapy available for the patient?
3 What are the symptoms of raised intracranial pressure?
4 Describe briefly the three methods of measuring intracranial pressure.
5 What hazards, for the patient, are associated with this technique?
6 What briefly is the medical treatment of raised intracranial pressure?

8

Respiratory Monitoring

The human body faces constant threat to its survival, from within itself and from the external environment. The effects that these hazards pose have physical consequences, none of which are more vital than those affecting the respiratory system. To help counteract these potential hazards the body has many intrinsic fail-safe mechanisms which defend vital organs and promote survival. In the critically ill patient many of these fail-safe mechanisms are activated, yet it may be necessary to augment or override them to preserve life.

The respiratory system responds rapidly, increasing or decreasing its capacity to compensate for changes in the internal or external environment. There are many instances when artificial ventilation must be used to control the effects of altered respiratory function, to preserve life and ensure recovery.

Intermittent Positive Pressure Ventilation (IPPV), is a technique by which lung function can be manipulated to optimize tissue perfusion and control to some extent the effects of systemic disease. Further consideration of IPPV will be given later in the chapter following a resumé of respiratory physiology.

The body has a number of basic needs, one of these is oxygen which is needed for effective metabolism of food, the end product of which is heat and energy. This is described as an aerobic process. Lack of oxygen causes anaerobic metabolism in which large quantities of lactic acid are produced, which compromise normal functions as it causes the blood pH to fall, cardiac function, inhibits enzyme activity and contributes to the breakdown of cell membranes.

The respiratory tract is divided into the upper and lower

sections, the upper section extending from the nose to the bronchioles is primarily concerned with mechanical movement of air from the atmosphere to the alveolus.

The larynx is an irregular shaped cartilaginous tube, continuous with the trachea which contains the vocal cords. It has a number of functions including voice production and efficient coughing. The cough reflex is produced by a build up of air within the thorax and forced expulsion of this air against the closed glottis.

The trachea is a large fibromuscular tube extending from the lower end of the larynx to the sternal angle, it is strengthened by C-shaped cartilaginous rings. At the level of the sternal angle the trachea divides into the left and right bronchi, which further sub-divide to serve the segmental lobes of each lung, (see Figure 8.1). The trachea and bronchi are lined with a ciliated mucous membrane which aids the removal of the debris from the lower segments of the lung tissue. The cilia acts as an 'escalator' forcing the debris upwards towards the larynx for expulsion. The right lung has three distinct lobes and the left two.

The right main bronchus is shorter and wider than the left, and enters the lung at a less acute angle this explains why during endotracheal intubation the right lung is more vulnerable to incorrect positioning of the tube into the right main bronchus. If not corrected this will cause collapse of the left lung as it will not be effectively ventilated. The walls of the bronchi contain Beta-2 sympathetic nerve receptors, these relax the tone of the airway when stimulated, causing dilation. The upper respiratory tract contains air which does not contribute to gaseous exchange, consequently this is referred to as dead space, the average amount for an adult being 150 ml. The dead space ensures carbon dioxide is not totally removed from the body during respiration, as a small amount is necessary to stimulate respiration and maintain vascular tone.

The bronchioles further subdivide and terminate in alveolar ducts which merge with alveolar sacs. The alveolus is one part of the alveolar sac, it is a thin walled balloon-like structure surrounded externally by capillaries. The alveoli have walls one cell thick, which are called pneumocytes. Gaseous exchange occurs across the alveolar membrane with oxygen

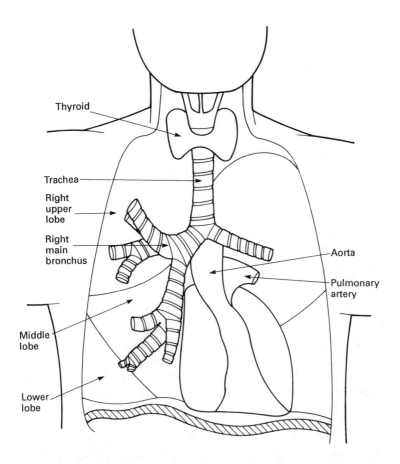

Figure 8.1   *Diagram showing the relationship between the intrathoracic structures.*

entering the capillary circulation while carbon dioxide moves in the opposite direction.

The alveolar cells produce pulmonary surfactant, this is a lipoprotein which reduces surface tension within the alveolus.

This prevents the alveolus collapsing during expiration, although if insufficient air is available, collapse may still occur. Macrophages are present within the alveolus, these cells can migrate through the alveolar wall and are phagocytic.

The blood supply to the alveoli is from the pulmonary artery. Blood is supplied separately to the bronchi and lung tissue from the bronchial arteries.

NORMAL INSPIRATION

Inspiration is an active process. Downward movement of the diaphragm causes an increase in lung volume. The intercostal muscles supplement this by raising the thoracic cage upwards and outward. The effect of the increased volume within the chest is to lower the pressure below atmospheric causing air to be sucked into the lungs.

The pleura enclose the lungs and lie in close proximity to the rib cage. It consists of two membranes, the parietal and visceral membranes. During inspiration the pleura adhere closely to the lungs.

Expiration

Expiration is a passive movement, in which the elastic recoil of the lungs, diaphragm and rib cage reduces the size of the thorax and forces air out of the chest under positive pressure. Where inflation of the chest, with air, is insufficient the accessory muscles are used signifying respiratory distress.

Lung Volumes

The lungs have a finite ability to expand, although their capacity exceeds the body's usual requirements for air, this is termed the functional residual capacity. Normal breathing involves only a percentage of lung capacity. Tidal volume measured in millilitres is the amount of air inspired and expired at each breath. Minute volume is the amount of air breathed in one minute and is measured in litres.

Vital capacity is the measurement of the total amount of air

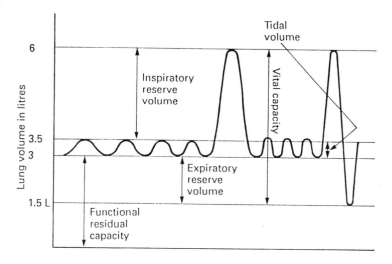

Figure 8.2   *Lung volumes.*

on maximum expiration following a maximum inspiration. Vital capacity, tidal volume and minute volumes are helpful indicators of respiratory function.

CONTROL OF RESPIRATION

The control mechanisms of respiration are within the brain tissue, stretch and chemoreceptors react to changes in the arterial pH, pCO_2 and pO_2 and stimulate the respiratory centre which modifies the breathing rate and volume. Inspired air contains a higher percentage of oxygen than does the blood in the pulmonary capillary. Therefore a diffusion gradient is present and oxygen diffuses down the gradient into the capillary. Conversely, carbon dioxide is present in higher concentrations in the capillary than the alveolus causing a diffusion gradient in the opposite direction to oxygen.

The pressure a gas exerts in a solution such as blood, is called the partial pressure or tension. The terms paO_2 and $paCO_2$ refer to the partial pressure of oxygen and carbon dioxide within arterial blood. It should be noted that the pressure exerted by a gas is dependent on its concentration, and is not affected by the presence of other gases.

Oxygen is carried bound to the protein haemoglobin (Hb), in the red blood cell, although a small percentage is carried in solution in the plasma. In normal physiology, the haemoglobin of oxygenated blood is 97% saturated with oxygen, and paO_2 is 100 mm Hg (13.3 kPa). If the partial pressure of oxygen falls then the oxygen saturation of Hb also falls, an important indication of hypoxia. The oxygen dissociation curve, (see Figure 8.3), demonstrates the relationship between partial pressure and Hb saturation.

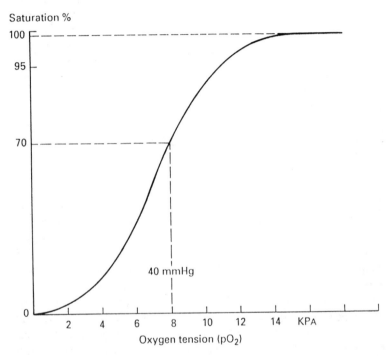

Figure 8.3 *Diagram of O_2 dissociation curve.*

Changes in paO_2 have a profound effect on Hb saturation. At a partial pressure of 40 mm Hg (5.3 kPa), for example, the Hb saturation falls to 70%. This may be insufficient to meet the oxygen demands of the tissues, although at low partial pressures Hb more readily gives up its oxygen. With high paO_2 levels the Hb becomes fully saturated, and is unable to carry more. Once the tissue needs for oxygen have been met there will be a surplus of unused oxygen which produces a slowing of the respiratory rate.

Changes within the pH of blood, body temperature and paO_2 will alter the haemoglobin's affinity for oxygen. This can be seen on the oxygen dissociation curve as a shift to the right or left. Movement of the curve to the right reduces Hb affinity for oxygen and encourages release of oxygen to the tissues. This can be caused by acidosis, hyperthermia, hypercarbia or hypoxia. Acidosis, in particular, causes the release of 2.3 diphosphoglycerate (DPG), an enzyme which reduces Hb affinity for oxygen, rapidly releasing it to the tissues. A left shift increases Hb affinity for oxygen and reduces diffusion of oxygen to the tissues. This is caused by a rise in pH, alkalaemia, hypothermia and hypocarbia. It can therefore be seen that delivery of the total quantity of oxygen, to the tissues, depends on three factors:

1 Cardiac output
2 The amount of available haemoglobin
3 The paO_2

Carbon dioxide (CO_2) is produced with water as a waste product of cell metabolism. As the CO_2 concentration in the cell exceeds that in the blood, carbon dioxide diffuses into the red blood cell, where it can be transported to the lungs (see Figure 8.4). The normal value of $paCO_2$ is 40 mm Hg (5.3 kPa). CO_2 enters the red blood cell, where the enzyme carbonic anhydrase, speeds up the dissolution of CO_2 to carbonic acid (H_2CO_3). At the same time oxygen is released from the red blood cell to the tissues, leaving behind the reduced or deoxygenated haemoglobin. The carbonic acid further dissociates to hydrogen ion (H^+) and bicarbonate ion (HCO_3^-) within the cell. The bicarbonate leaves the cell and enters the plasma. To maintain electrolyte equilibrium chloride ion (Cl^-) enters from the plasma. At this stage the red blood cell contains, chloride, potassium and reduced haemoglobin. When the blood cell reaches the lungs the process reverses, CO_2 is released and exchanged for oxygen.

Carbon dioxide can also be carried in solution in plasma, as well as attached to Hb in the cell. The attachment of CO_2 to Hb is at a different part of the Hb molecule to that of O_2.

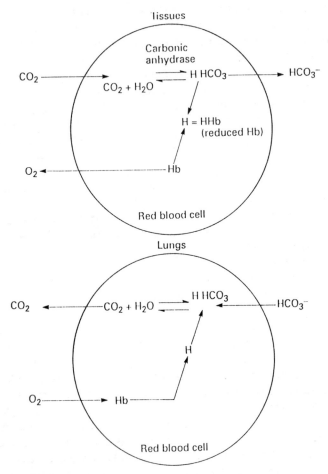

Figure 8.4 *Diagram showing the carriage of CO_2 from tissues to the lungs by red blood cells.*

MAINTENANCE OF pH

pH is the hydrogen ion balance of blood and other tissues fluids, and is the indicator of acidity or alkalinity. pH readings below the level of 7, indicate acid and above 7, alkali. The maintenance of cell membranes and enzyme activity is dependent on the control of pH within a small range. The normal pH of blood being 7.36–7.44.

The respiratory and renal systems strive to maintain blood pH within this narrow range. There are a number of mechanisms within the body which assist in the maintenance of constant pH. These include:

1 Kidneys: The kidneys produce a buffer solution of bicarbonate, HCO_3^- which can be used to mop up free acids. This HCO_3^- formation takes place within the renal tubule cells.

2 Lungs: the lungs alter their activity in response to changes in pH. Alkalaemia causing, reduction in respiratory rate and volume. The effect of this being an increase in CO_2 levels. CO_2 retention makes the blood more acid and reduces the high level of the pH. Decreased pH causes increased breathing, and hence reduces the CO_2 level of the blood, causing a rise in the pH back to near normal levels.

3 Plasma proteins and Hb: These proteins can mop up either acid or alkali. This buffers the effect of these substances on the blood pH for a short time.

4 Other chemical reactions, to a lesser extent, remove hydrogen and hydroxyl ions from the blood and help to maintain the pH.

It can be seen that respiration is a finely balanced mechanism which is highly responsive to changes in the internal and external environment.

INTERMITTENT POSITIVE PRESSURE VENTILATION (IPPV)

Despite the many different makes of ventilators available, these machines can be roughly divided into two groups, pressure generators and volume generators. Each group generates air flow to inflate the lungs at inspiration, and then cycle to expiration, which is a passive process.

Two main factors influence the type of ventilator used:

1 Lung compliance: This is the elasticity of the lungs. The greater the force needed to inflate the lungs, the lower the compliance. Respiratory diseases in particular cause reduced lung compliance and increased difficulty in breathing for the patient.

2 Airway resistance: The airways have a limited ability to stretch. Partial occlusion of the airway, by secretions, inflammation etc, will increase the resistance to the flow of

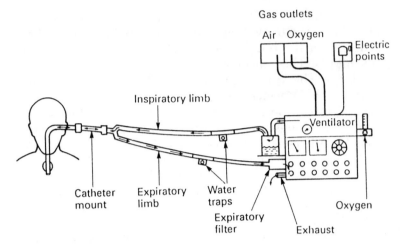

Figure 8.5 *Diagram showing a ventilator circuit.*

gas. Asthma, is a good example of increased airway resistance.

The type of ventilator selected will therefore have to meet the patient's needs and be capable of ventilating the patient satisfactorily, taking into account the possible difficulties imposed by lung compliance and airway resistance.

Pressure Generators

These ventilators generate a pre-set airway pressure. Once reached the machine cycles to expiration, the gas flow stops and the patient can breathe out using the elastic recoil of the lung tissue, ribs and diaphragm. This type of ventilation may be unsuited to patients with decreased compliance or increased airway resistance, as the pre-set pressure is reached very quickly causing a reduced tidal and minute volume to be delivered.

Volume Generators

Volume or flow generators deliver a pre-set volume, which is unaffected by lung compliance or airway resistance. These ventilators generate sufficient power to force the pre-set gas flow into the lungs regardless of compliance or airway pressure. Some volume generators cycle to expiration at a pre-set time. Volume generators are used in most specialized units as pre-set tidal and minute volumes are delivered regardless of lung changes.

Ventilator Modes

Increasing sophistication of ventilators permits different modes of ventilation to be used, this ensures the patients comfort and optimizes the effect of ventilatory therapy. The ventilator can be used in two main ways:

- As a controller, in which the patient is prevented from making any contribution to their own breathing, this usually necessitates the patient being heavily sedated.
- As an assistor, in which the patient's breathing is augmented by the ventilator. Alteration in the ventilator mode can optimize oxygenation and permit a more 'normal' type of breathing, which will be more acceptable to the patient.

Specifically some of the more frequently used modes are as follows.

Mandatory Ventilation, Controller Mode

This mode of ventilation is used in a limited number of patients. The ventilator is pre-set to deliver a predetermined minute volume. The patient usually needs to be heavily sedated to prevent them from fighting to breathe against the ventilator. Large amounts of sedative drugs may be needed to obtain patient acquiescence, an unsatisfactory situation, as metabolism and excretion of these drugs may be prolonged in the seriously ill patient. This mode of ventilation should only be used in situations where control of ventilation and maintenance of blood gases is paramount, i.e. severe hypoxaemia.

Pressure Support, Assist Mode

Pressure support provides a continuous gas flow during the whole cycle of breathing. A small positive pressure is pre-set to be delivered on inspiration, this acts as a boost to inspiration. An analogy would be, the lung resembles a balloon, and like a balloon, inflation from the collapsed state is difficult. As the balloon receives more air, it increases in size and inflation then becomes progressively easier. Initially the fibres in the walls of the balloon are close together and therefore form a strong bond. As the volume of the balloon increases the fibres move further apart, making them less able to cling together, reducing resistance to inflation. At low levels pressure support minimizes breathing effort and at high levels improves tidal volume. This mode can be used in conjunction with others, i.e. pressure support and SIMV.

Mandatory Minute Volume (MMV), Assist Mode

Mandatory minute volume ventilation (MMV) is used to wean the patient from IPPV by automatically reducing ventilator minute volume as spontaneous breathing increases. The ventilator monitors the patient's breathing pattern and intervenes only if the pre-set minute volume is not met, by delivering a tidal volume.

Synchronized Intermittent Mandatory Ventilation (SIMV), Assist Mode

The patient receives pre-set mandatory respirations, in the periods between these mandatory respirations, they can take spontaneous unassisted respirations. Synchronization of the ventilator ensures mandatory breaths are not delivered at inappropriate times, i.e. during expiration. This method of ventilation permits control of arterial blood gas tensions, whilst ensuring exercise of respiratory muscles and patient comfort.

Intermittent Mandatory Ventilation (IMV), Assist Mode

This mode is similar to SIMV, in that the mandatory respiratory rate is reduced slowly to permit the patient to take progressively more spontaneous respirations. As the mode is unsynchronized, the mandatory respirations may be delivered during expiration, this can prove very unpleasant for the patient and makes this mode less effective than SIMV.

Trigger, Assist Mode

The ventilator can be made sensitive to the patient's desire to breathe. By attempting to take a breath, the patient creates a negative intrathoracic pressure, which is sensed by the machine. The machine responds to this negative pressure by delivering a tidal volume to the patient. The sensitivity of the trigger mechanism can be varied, making it either more difficult or easier for the patient to take a breath. The trigger device is also important as it aids the patient in coughing. Coughing can only occur if air is present in the chest, and the patient has a negative intrathoracic pressure.

MMV, SIMV and trigger are all modes of ventilation which can be used to wean patients from IPPV to spontaneous respiration. By selecting the correct mode of ventilation, patient comfort, effective ventilation and maintenance of blood gases can be achieved.

Endotracheal Intubation

To facilitate IPPV an endotracheal tube is inserted through the larynx and into the trachea. The tube, made of light plastic has a balloon, cuff, attached to its lower outside end. The cuff can be inflated to occlude the trachea and prevent air escaping the chest around the outside of the tube. The cuff also prevents aspiration of secretions and vomitus into the chest from the upper tract. The correct size of tube is 7–8 mm for women and 8–9 mm for men. The mm measurement refers to the internal diameter of the tube.

The endotracheal tube can be inserted nasally or orally. Oral intubation is preferred in emergency situations, as the technique is often easier to perform. The disadvantages of this technique are excessive movement and potential occlusion of the tube, due to manipulation by the patient's tongue or teeth, difficulty with lip-reading and increased salivation. Ulceration and infection of the mouth occur due to difficulties in performing oral toilet. Oral intubation may also be precluded in patients with maxillo facial injuries.

Nasal tubes are often preferred by the patient, as the nose provides more support for the tube and restricts its movement.

The patient can often swallow more easily. Oral hygiene and lip-reading are facilitated. Nasal intubation is a more difficult technique to perform as the tube may have to be manipulated into place by forceps and an introducer. The patient's cardiovascular system must be stable enough to withstand this slightly prolonged procedure. Other disadvantages of the technique include the potential risk of sinusitis and trauma to the nasal mucosa. Nasal tubes also tend to kink more easily, partially occluding the lumen, as the nasal tube tends to be longer and narrower than the oral tube. A chest X-ray must be performed following intubation to check that the tube is correctly positioned.

Excessive and prolonged pressure of the inflated cuff on the tracheal wall causes reduction of capillary blood flow to that portion of the trachea. This may cause ulceration, scar tissue formation and stenosis. The high volume, low pressure cuffs help to prevent this, it is mainly a problem with the red rubber endotracheal tubes. Small, portable cuff pressure monitors are available. These monitors measure the cuff pressure, as resistance to inflation, permitting correct filling and maintenance of a safe pressure within the cuff. If large quantities of air are required to achieve a seal then the tube may be too small.

If a pressure monitor is unavailable, the cuff should be gently inflated with air until gurgling or hissing sounds, heard on patient expiration are abolished. These sounds are due to air escaping around the partially inflated cuff, their disappearance therefore indicates the cuff is correctly inflated. The amount of air required to achieve a seal and the size of the entrotracheal tube should be documented.

Whatever methods are used to secure the tube into position, it is important that the tape used is not elastic and that the angles of the mouth and ears are protected from chaffing. Soiled tapes must be changed frequently to reduce the risk of infection and ensure patient comfort.

Endotracheal intubation prevents effective coughing and expectoration. Aspiration of sputum must be performed to maintain airway patency, ensure patient comfort and reduce airway resistance. Poor suction technique and unclean equipment, predisposes the patient to nosocomial infection. The suction technique should therefore be performed as a sterile procedure.

Humidification

The upper airway normally warms, moistens and filters air, intubation bypasses this. Breathing dry gas is unpleasant, it causes dehydration and increases the tenacity of secretions. It is therefore important that the intubated patient breathes humidified gas.

Water bath humidifiers can be used in the breathing circuit. The inspiratory gases flow through the warmed water and are humidified. The gas is saturated with water vapour at a temperature of 55-60 degrees centigrade and inhaled (see Figure 8.6).

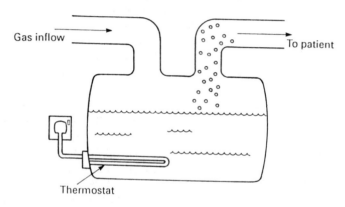

Figure 8.6   *Water bath humidifier with immersion heater.*

Nebulizers are fluid filled containers in which a high pressure gas supply enters through a small port. Water is drawn through a second port and is vaporized by the gas flow. The force of the gas flow forms a saturated fine mist which is then inhaled. Nebulizers are much more efficient than humidifiers, but the gas flow must be closely observed to ensure the nebulizer is functioning efficiently.

Condensation in the breathing circuit collects and must be removed frequently, to prevent obstruction to inspiration, and prevent accidental aspiration of water into the patient's chest. As a further precaution the breathing circuit must always be positioned lower than the patient's head.

All equipment used in respiratory therapy is prone to bacterial colonization. Where possible disposable single patient use items can help to reduce the risks of cross infection.

Nursing Role

Following establishment of ventilation the nurse should take the opportunity to assess and monitor patient response to this procedure. IPPV is often used to correct hypoxaemia or ventilatory failure, the seriousness of the diagnosis makes close observation imperative.

Hypoxaemia causes restlessness, confusion, sweating and hyperventilation. If severe the patient may be stuporose or in coma. Cyanosis may not be seen until the paO_2 falls below 50 mm Hg (6.7 kPa). Hypercarbia causes drowsiness, confusion and stupor. The patient's limbs may feel warm, and bounding pulses are present due to the vasodilator effect of CO_2.

As part of the assessment the nurse should observe the oral mucosa for signs of cyanosis. The patient's skin should also be observed for signs of cyanosis and hypercarbia. The presence of cold clammy skin indicates shock which must be immediately reported.

Following intubation the patient should have a chest X-ray to confirm correct positioning of the endotracheal tube. It should be remembered that movement of the tube either into the right main bronchus, or an upward displacement through the vocal cords may occur following patient movement or insecure taping of the endotracheal tube. By observing the patient's chest movement and to some extent the patients compliance the nurse can check that both sides of the chest move together and that the breathing pattern conforms to the ventilator settings. Observations of chest movements are best performed at the end of the bed, where both sides of the chest can be visualized and compared more easily. Increased inflation of one side of the chest, or paradoxical chest movements, may indicate a dislodged endotracheal tube, pneumothorax or flail chest segment. Also listen for breath sounds with a stethoscope.

In the early stages after ventilation is commenced, the patient's compliance to ventilation should be assessed. Sweating, patient distress and attempts to breathe indicate that the patient is uncomfortable, and that ventilation is inadequate.

Fighting the ventilator imposes severe strain on the patient, it increases oxygen demand, cardiac workload and provokes hypercarbia. The psychological effects of this situation may also affect patient recovery time and morale.

The nurse must also observe that the endotracheal tube and ventilator circuit remain patent. Obstruction or disconnection of the tubing can occur at any time, or at any point between the patient and the ventilator. The endotracheal tube may become obstructed with secretions, or by the patient biting the tube. The position of the patient's head may also cause the tube to kink, obstructing the gas flow. The nurse should ensure that each connection is patent and secure and that condensed water vapour and secretions are cleared frequently. The ventilator circuit tubing must be correctly positioned and supported and the ventilator alarms switched on.

Endotracheal intubation and IPPV prevents effective coughing and expectoration. The presence of endotracheal tubes may also act as an irritant to the trachea causing excessive coughing and gagging by the patient. Gross movement of the tube will also provoke coughing. Care must be taken not to move the tube unduly, either during suctioning or whilst performing other duties.

The tracheal secretions give important information about the patient's condition. Specimens of sputum should be routinely taken for microbiological examination. Endotracheal intubation effectively by-passes many of the defense mechanisms in the upper respiratory tract, and may leave the patient prone to infection. The colour and consistency of the secretions are also indicators of the onset of complications, i.e. pulmonary oedema, and should therefore be reported and documented.

Careful observation of the patient will help the nurse to provide a good standard of care, and permit prompt treatment of potentially dangerous and unpleasant complications.

MONITORING AND ASSESSING VENTILATOR SETTINGS

The ventilator settings are manipulated to suit the patient's needs and to optimize respiratory function. The nurse's role is to closely observe and intervene as appropriate to maintain the patient's safety and comfort. The nurse must be familiar with the function of the ventilator settings to ensure potential problems are anticipated. A brief resumé of the ventilator functions and settings follows.

Minute Volume

The expired minute volume is measured in litres. Changes in the reading, obtained from the ventilator, may indicate either a leak of gas, if the reading is low, or excessive patient breathing if the reading is higher than set. If a leak in the patient circuit is suspected, the patient must be manually ventilated as the source of the leak may take some time to isolate. As well as checking the security of all the connections and emptying the tubing of water, the gas inflow pipes must be checked to ensure they have not been kinked or compressed by other equipment.

Airway Pressure

The airway pressure rises and falls with inspiration and expiration. This meter measures the force of gas necessary to inflate the chest with air. A low pressure reading may indicate a leak in the circuit or improvement in the lung compliance. A raised reading indicates increased resistance to gas flow and may be due to a number of factors, including condensed water in the circuit, obstruction of the airways by sputum or the obstruction of the endotracheal tube due to the patient biting it. Progressive rises in airway pressure may be due to deteriorating lung compliance infection, oedema or pneumothorax. The cause must be detected and treated quickly. Doubts about the efficiency of the ventilator should be acted upon rapidly.

Frequency

The ventilator rate may be displayed on a dial, although some ventilators do not have a rate meter and the rate of breaths must be counted manually. For those using machines with rate dials, it is good practice to occasionally count the breath rate manually to check the accuracy of the machine.

Inspiratory/Expiratory Ratio (I/E Ratio)

Most ventilators have a fixed I/E ratio. This ratio refers to the time set for inspiration and expiration. The normal I/E ratio is one second for inspiration and two seconds for expiration, giving an I/E ratio of 1:2. In some cases the I:E ratio can be manipulated to optimize oxygenation. This may take the form of prolonging the expiratory time to three or more seconds. This is useful, for example, in patients with asthma who have difficulty breathing out, due to bronchospasm. By prolonging expiratory time the patient has a longer period for gaseous exchange, which helps to maintain their paO_2. It is important to ensure the I/E ratio is correctly set, not all patients benefit from a lengthened expiratory time.

Positive End Expiratory Pressure (PEEP)

Positive end expiratory pressure is a resistance applied during expiration. This prevents collapse of the alveoli during expiration, thus prolonging the time available for gaseous exchange, improving oxygenation. The normal range of PEEP used is +2 to +15 cm of water, although in some cases higher pressures can be used. The procedure has disadvantages however. Continuous positive pressure within the chest suppresses the thoracic pump and reduces blood flow into the right side of the heart, resulting in reduced cardiac output and inaccurate CVP readings, PEEP accentuates this problem. There is also an increased risk of pneumothorax when PEEP is used.

Oxygen Entrainment

The inspired oxygen percentage can be altered to meet each patient's needs. It is important that the oxygen percentage is checked with an oxygen analyser to ensure correct oxygen percentage is administered. Greater than 80% oxygen for longer than 24/48 hours can lead to permanent damage to lung tissue (fibrosis).

Physiological Effects of IPPV

1 Increased mean airway pressure, and airway resistance.
2 Increased mean intrathoracic pressure and decreased venous return into the right side of the heart.
3 Decreased cardiac output.
4 a Initial increase in sympathetic tone, causing tachycardia, hypertension and increased myocardial contractility, then:
   b Decrease in vascular tone, hypovolaemia, reduced heart rate and reduced myocardial contractile force.
5 Increased intracranial pressure, due to decreased venous return from the jugular veins.
6 Diminished urine output due to the effects of reduced cardiac output on the renal blood flow.
7 Decreased effort of breathing.
8 Increased dead space ventilation, and increased ventilation of the apices of the lungs in preference to the bases. Blood flow to the bases of the lungs is increased, giving rise to a mismatch of ventilation and perfusion. This causes shunting of blood through the pulmonary circulation, seriously affecting the paO_2 and $paCO_2$.
9 Incorrect ventilator settings may cause hyper/hypo ventilation which in turn, causes serious alteration to the blood gas tensions, leading to respiratory acidosis/alkalosis.
10 Increased gastric secretions and stress ulceration of the stomach lining may result from IPPV, which also increases intra-abdominal pressure resulting in a decrease in gut motility and possible paralytic ileus.

Air swallowing is a common feature of ventilated patients, this may cause dilation of the stomach, splinting of the diaphragm and colic.

PSYCHOLOGICAL EFFECTS

Termed sensory deprivation or overload, this situation is characterized by feelings of fear, apprehension, isolation and anxiety. Insomnia, frustration and depression may also present as symptoms. Dependence on the ventilator may also develop making the task of restoring spontaneous respiration more difficult. These factors are dealt with in the final chapter in detail.

Arterial Blood Gas Sampling

Arterial blood gas samples enable close observation of respiratory function and maintenance of blood pH. Serial sampling shows important trends in the patient's response to therapy.

The blood gas analyser gives a range of results, the important ones being pH, pCO_2, pO_2, SBC (Standard Bicarbonate), base excess and saturation %. Analysis of these results permits manipulation of IPPV or oxygen therapy, to suit the patients needs.   When interpreting arterial blood gas results the nurse should observe the results in sequence, i.e.:

1 pH: Is it normal, acidotic or alkalotic?
2 pCO_2: Is it normal, increased or decreased?
3 SBC: Is it normal, increased or decreased?
4 Base Excess (BE): Is it positive, negative or within the normal range?. Base excess refers to the amount of alkali buffer available in the blood. If the blood becomes acidotic buffers mop up the acid and return the pH to normal. By adding buffer to the blood, the stores of buffer are depleted leading to a base deficit, a negative reading. In alkalosis, acid must be added to the blood to return the pH to normal. The alkali buffer is untouched and remains as base excess, a positive reading.
5 pO_2 and saturation %: Is it normal, increased or decreased?

The following examples show some changes in pH, pCO_2 and HCO_3^- which may occur with respiratory and metabolic alkalosis.

The normal values are:

pH:	7.36–7.44
pCO_2:	35–40 mm Hg (5.3–5.9 kPa)
SBC (Standard Bicarbonate):	22–26 mmol/litre
BE (Base Excess):	−2–+2 mmol/litre

Examples

Reading		*Analysis*
pH	7.20	Low
pCO_2	70 (9.3)	High
SBC	22	Normal
BE	0	Normal

In this example SBC and BE are normal which indicates that the raised pCO_2 is of respiratory origin – **Respiratory Acidosis**

Reading		*Analysis*
pH	7.5	High
pCO_2	30 (4)	Low
SBC	24	Normal
BE	+2	Normal

In this example the bicarbonate and BE are normal, the pH is deranged and the pCO_2 is low indicating – **Respiratory Alkalosis**

Reading		*Analysis*
pH	7.23	Low
pCO_2	26 (3.4)	Low
SBC	18	Low
BE	−14	Negative

The low pH indicates acidosis. The low pCO_2 indicates that respiration is not the cause of the acidosis. The low bicarbonate and BE indicate the origin is metabolic – **Metabolic Acidosis.**

Reading		*Analysis*
pH	7.52	High
pCO_2	40 (5.3)	Normal
SBC	43	High
BE	+10	Positive

The high pH and normal pCO_2 indicates the alkalosis is metabolic in origin – **Metabolic Alkalosis.**

In certain situations the blood pH will be maintained within normal limits at the expense of the pCO_2, SBC and BE. By maintaining the pH the situation is said to be compensated for. Such a situation usually does not require treatment, rather close monitoring to ensure that the pH remains normal and that the body can continue to cope. Investigations as to the cause of this compensated state should also commence.

Results of blood gas analysis may alter both the medical and nursing care given to the patient.

1 Respiratory acidosis indicates deterioration of respiratory function. IPPV may be required to control the effects of this acidosis and support the patient until recovery occurs.

2 Respiratory alkalosis may be caused by hyper or over ventilation which can be corrected by reduction in the ventilatory volume and/or rate. Over breathing, is not confined to the ventilated patient, and may be due to fear, pain or anxiety.

3 Metabolic acidosis may be caused by a number of disease processes including diabetes mellitus and septicaemia. The cause of the acidosis should be treated as well as the effects.

4 Metabolic alkalosis is difficult to treat. It may be due to loss of gastric acid, vomiting and administration of sodium bicarbonate. Potassium depletion may also lead to alkalosis. Potassium replacement therapy will correct this type of alkalosis.

Arterial blood specimens may be taken via an established arterial cannula or as an isolated arterial puncture, with a heparinized syringe and needle. This latter procedure is performed by medical staff. The sample may be taken from either of the radial or femoral arteries. As discussed in Chapter 5, the presence of a collateral circulation should be confirmed prior to taking the sample. The puncture site must be compressed for at least five minutes following sampling, and the site checked frequently for signs of bleeding or haematoma.

Mistakes in interpreting blood gas results may be caused by a number of factors:

- Delay in processing the sample
- High patient temperature
- Anaemia
- Samples taken following sodium bicarbonate or large blood transfusion
- Over breathing whilst sample being taken

Acid base is an important physiological function. Understanding of the results of blood gas analysis can ensure appropriate treatment, of potential life-threatening situations, is given promptly and nursing care can be adapted to anticipate and cater for the patients needs.

RESPIRATION — EXERCISES

1 Why is it necessary for the blood pH to be maintained within the narrow range of 7.36–7.44?
2 What role do the kidneys play in the maintenance of blood pH?
3 What do you understand by the term lung compliance?
4 What do you understand by the term controlled ventilation?
5 List the advantages and disadvantages of nasal intubation.
6 How is inspired gas humidified?
7 List five physiological effects of artificial ventilation.
8 What mistakes can be made interpreting blood gas results?

9

Effects of Monitoring

Open the door into any Intensive Care Unit (ITU) and the first thing to catch your eye are the machines. Usually they are stacked close together, with lights flashing and occasionally alarms sounding. Somewhere in the midst of it all is the patient. Ask any staff new to ITU, what worries or frightens them most and the answer invariably is 'the machines'. This is not altogether a surprising reaction! Interestingly though, in recent years, our society has been revolutionized by the impact of computers and the seemingly endless uses for the micro-chip. Yet our responses to complex machinery tends to be negative in the first instance. This response is often aggravated by fear, anxiety and ignorance.

The equipment used in the care of the critically ill patient allows prompt diagnosis and treatment of potential crisis. That is why it is there. Despite the frightening appearance of all this hi-tech gadgetry, the nurse must never lose sight of this simple fact, or of the patient connected to the array of monitoring equipment.

EFFECTS OF MONITORING ON THE PATIENT

Admission to hospital for any reason is a traumatic event. Quite apart from the stress caused by an illness or injury, the sudden change in role, with a heavy accent on dependence causes innumerable problems of adjustment. The unfamiliar environment, changed routine and isolation from family and friends for large parts of the day intensify feelings of stress and anxiety. Self esteem and feelings of worth are affected. Fear and loneliness are exacerbated by pain and discomfort.

Further stressors, such as the various monitoring techniques, compound feelings of anxiety and distress. Physiological changes may exacerbate psychological distress. Reduction in cardiac output, imbalance of arterial blood gas tensions and administration of drugs for example, serve to confuse and disorientate the patient.

It is important to note that not all patients admitted to ITU are intubated, ventilated and unconscious, although those that are often experience the most acute and traumatic psychological effects. Admission may also be on the grounds of close and frequent monitoring. In the situation where the patient is intubated and ventilated, control of the patient's body is taken away from them. The realization by the patient that they have lost control over their body and environment, understandably leads to feelings such as low morale, apathy or anxiety. It should also be remembered that pain also tends to lower self esteem. Low morale has a detrimental effect on the patient's recovery, as they feel unable to make appropriate decisions, and the patient may effectively resist efforts to encourage a degree of independence.

Fear is a major part of the ITU patient's life, fear of discomfort, pain, or death added to worries about home contributing to the patient's distress. Loss of interest in the outside world, preoccupation with physical health, and irritability are typical signs of intense anxiety and increased stress.

Sleep disturbances are common in ITU, in particular loss of REM sleep (Rapid Eye Movement). REM sleep is thought to influence thinking and problem solving, and occurs several times per night. As the name implies REM sleep is associated with rapid eye movements and dreaming. Sleep deprivation and its effects are difficult to quantify. Experiments by Gulevich et al in 1966 and McGaugh et al in 1979, failed to show any serious consequences, even in sleep deprivation of up to five days. A rebound effect tends to occur following a period of sleeplessness, REM sleep increasing in the following recovery period. The main consequences of sleep disturbance or deprivation, appears to be drowsiness, increased desire to sleep, and a tendency to fall asleep easily. Experiments by Webb in 1975 and Dement in 1976 cite inattention to detail, minor confusions and misconceptions, but no seriously disturbed behaviour. However it must be presumed that these experiments were carried out on subjects who were not in ill health.

In many patients, frequent disturbance and over stimulation, by medical and nursing procedures can result in psychological problems. Prolonged stays in ITU offer no opportunity for catching up on sleep and may combine with other factors to produce disturbed behaviour patterns. If sleep patterns are disturbed, so too are circadian rhythms. Circadian rhythms ensure peak efficiency of body function during the day and a rest and recovery period at night. These rhythms act in a similar way to a clock, the whole cycle lasting for approximately 25 hours. Like the heart rate each individuals body clock is unique. Although length of sleep can be varied at will, or by alarm clock, other bodily functions remain on a less variable time basis. Circadian rhythms have been shown to govern body temperature, urine excretion, hormonal secretion, cell division and enzyme synthesis. Disruption of the body clock may alter all these factors. Changes in mood, judgement ability and cognitive skills are also affected. At certain times within the cycle, of 25 hours, vulnerability to pain, endotoxin, infection and medications are increased. Allergic reactions may also occur when the cycle is in the resting mode, i.e. late evening/early morning.

Desynchronization of the circadian rhythm affects us all. Shift patterns, in particular night duty, are a well known cause of disturbed circadian rhythms in nurses. Diurnal rhythms are the bodily responses to the passage of time, i.e. day and night. The human body is programmed to be awake during the day, with a peak in performance at about midday. Each of us has functions and tasks to perform each day. To enable us to meet and deal effectively with such stresses, the body releases hormones, optimizes muscle function by increasing cardiac output, releasing adequate nutrients and oxygen, and heightens our awareness and perception. These responses ensure our maximum performance is attainable as needed. At the end of each day however rest and recovery is necessary to ensure our continued health.

To a certain extent reduction of light combined with physical sensations of fatigue induce a slowing of our responses, a winding down period prior to sleep in the evening. The patient in the ITU may be deprived of the ability to respond to changes in time. Lights may be left on for long periods, so that the patient is unaware of whether it is day or night, the level of noise may not decrease and without a visible clock the patient quickly loses track of time. Continued disturbance to measure various parameters denies the patient sleep. The result may be confusion of the 'body clock' causing in some cases a complete reversal of sleep patterns, i.e. insomnia at night and drowsiness during the day. The situation is further exacerbated if the unit has no windows or the beds are arranged in such a way that the patients are unable to see the windows that are there. Day and night loses all meaning and adds to confusion and disorientation.

Sensory deprivation is another feature which contributes to confusion and misperception for the critically ill patient. In the patient receiving maximum monitoring and supportive therapies (i.e. IPPV, Swan Ganz monitoring, intravenous infusions, etc) a certain degree of immobility is enforced. The patient's arms, head and legs may be bandaged or otherwise restricted by splints and tubes, and movement may be inhibited by pain. This immobility provokes a number of problems for a patient, the only available stimuli may be the touch of the sheets, monotonous and unidentified sounds and the sudden movement of people into and out of their peripheral vision. Human contact is dramatically reduced, and the presence of endotracheal tubes makes vocal communication impossible. Spectacles and hearing aids may not be available. The whole being compounded by staff who do not engage in meaningful communication with the patient, a common criticism of ITU staff in the past.

The patient is totally vulnerable, unable to speak, and in particular, call for help, unable to focus or hear properly and immobile with no sense of day or night. Research with fit and well volunteers has shown how only 24 hours sensory deprivation is sufficient to produce hallucinations, confusion, paranoia and severe anxiety. The message for the nurse is clear, despite all the monitoring equipment, communicate with the patient, give them sensory input they can understand. Severe psychological distress can be avoided in this way.

Sensory overload is a term used to explain the vast amount of physical and psychological stimuli which may be received by some patients. This is not unlike sensory deprivation in its effects. The patient is bombarded by stimuli from many sources. Medical and nursing procedures, frequently related to monitoring, may be virtually constant, particularly in the patient whose condition is unstable. A multiplicity of alien sounds, sudden unexplained noises, such as machine alarms, and the general hubbub of the unit contribute to the effects of pain, hypoxia, hypercarbia, drugs and reduced cardiac output.

Both sensory deprivation and overload produce symptoms which have been variously described as the ITU psychosis/syndrome, or more colloquially as white walls, or white walling. The patient is anxious, restless, confused and distressed. Disorientation to time and place occurs. The patient may experience intense and conflicting emotions including frustration, anger, anxiety, apathy, depression and in some cases paranoid thoughts. These emotions alternate rapidly from one to another like a roller coaster ride. The patient's sense of security and personal value is undermined, leaving them distressed, anxious and feeling very vulnerable and with low morale. Delusional thoughts and hallucinations are common and have been well documented. A common delusion is the patients misplaced conception of where they are. Many feel they are not in hospital at all but at home perhaps, or in prison, in a foreign country or in some surreal place. For example patients may imagine themselves to be in another country, they may appear not to understand any request or information given them. Only later does it become evident that they thought themselves in a foreign country and unable to speak the language there.

Intensive care units by definition are busy places and patients are nursed in close proximity to each other. Privacy may be at a premium. Adequate observation necessitates a clear field of vision for the nurse. Screens and curtains may be inadequate and invariably the patient is nursed naked. The seemingly asleep patient can easily be ignored. Examination of the patient without explanation and with little regard for the patient's privacy and feelings may be a feature of the inexperienced and uninitiated to ITU.

Conversations not involving the patient, but within their hearing may be misconstrued. Staff talking perhaps about other patients may forget the patient may be listening and may interpret their comments as relating to themselves. Apparently unconscious patients have frequently given very accurate accounts of conversations at their bedside, subsequently. It is better to think of such patients as unresponsive, they may be very conscious of what is being said around them.

For the patient not sedated and able to communicate, psychological problems may also occur. Isolation, introspection and increased dependence on hospital staff may give rise to demanding and difficult behaviour. The patient may be unable to see or appreciate the realities of the situation they find themselves in. The increased ratio of staff to patients means that in most situations nurses are allocated to patients on a 1:1 basis. The patient is initially encouraged to relinquish their independence to ensure effective treatment. Once the presenting condition is controlled the patient has to be weaned from total dependence and encouraged to take up responsibility for their lives once again. Monitoring and hence nurse/patient interaction becomes less frequent. This removal of support may cause intense fear and feelings of lack of security. This may then present as demanding, aggressive and sometimes belligerent behaviour. This can have serious consequences following transfer, of the patient, to general wards. The patient feels less secure and less important. The display of demanding behaviour and an apparently unreasonable and sometimes hostile attitude can further alienate him/her from their peers and the carers. The patient is actually saying he/she is unhappy and frightened. This situation obviously will affect recovery rate and progress, and will colour the patient's future dealings with the hospital.

Nursing these patients demands endless patience and understanding. Unfortunately however this demanding behaviour tends to reinforce negative attitudes held by staff towards both the patient in particular and specialized units in general.

The presence of relatives and close friends can be reassuring. Relatives are a source of encouragement and comfort, they reduce sensations of isolation and bring news of home and family. If the patient is confused this may be preferable, to the relatives than no response at all.

As humans, we rely on the clues given to us by gestures, eye contact and verbal means to carry out effective communication. The lack of feedback from the sedated and immobile patient makes conversation difficult. The relatives, or the nurse, may feel inhibited and embarrassed about appearing to be talking to themselves, in a room full of strangers. A common response of some relatives to this situation is repeated entreaties to the patient to open their eyes when this is not possible. The real business of communication, such as passing on news, and conversation to the patient is consequently lost. It stands repeating that apparently unconscious patients should be thought of as unresponsive and communication should occur as though they can hear every word. The effects of altered tissue perfusion have been discussed in previous chapters, but must be mentioned as a contributory cause of confusion and disorientation.

Drug therapies within the ITU environment are major factors contributing to altered perception and consciousness. Sedation in its many forms alters the patient's perceptual abilities. Many of the analgesic drugs have the side effect of euphoria, and increase dreaming. These drugs are necessary for the patient's physical comfort and to facilitate painful or unpleasant procedures. Malfunction of the excretory organs, i.e. kidney, liver etc, may cause delayed excretion of the drugs, prolonging their effects. Some antibiotic and diuretic drugs may cause physical damage to tissues, such as large doses of diuretic drugs which can produce deafness. Aminoglycoside antibiotics are nephrotoxic, i.e. they are poisonous in large doses to the renal cells. Excretion of drugs, is a primary ability of the renal cells, damage to them will prevent effective excretion of many drugs, particularly the sedatives, which will in turn affect the patient's awareness and orientation.

The influence of the media has had a profound effect on the general public's awareness and expectations of medical advances, practices and treatments. Television almost daily, presents us with the opportunity to examine and closely scrutinize medical care. In programmes relating to hospital care, technical machinery is often much in evidence, cardiac monitors being frequently shown. Alterations in the waveforms are often used to provide dramatic effect. Despite this, use of equipment without adequate supporting information may reinforce misconceptions and inappropriate expectations. An example of this might be that the monitor is some way influences the patient's heart function. The function of the electrodes, used to facilitate monitoring may also be misunderstood. The electrodes may be viewed not as adhesive pads used to detect electrical activity through the skin, but as having the ability to affect cardiac function. They may be seen as in some way to be keeping the heart going. Sudden non-adherence of the electrodes inevitably causes alteration of the waveform and activation of the alarm. The consequences of the electrode falling off and the alarm sounding may therefore produce anxiety and fear both in the patient and in the relative. Without adequate information about monitor function and potential false alarms, both patient and relatives become apprehensive unnecessarily fearing cardiac dysfunction. Such dysfunctions can be associated with all monitoring equipment therefore adequate explanation is vital to prevent unnecessary anxiety.

In most specialized units the equipment tends to be located behind the bed head, and obscured from the patient's direct vision. The patient's attention may be drawn to it by automatic alarm activity but often they appear unaware and undisturbed by its presence. In circumstances where the patient is conscious and aware, the experience may be however, more positive. Complex monitoring equipment may give the patient both a sense of security and importance. Some patients and relatives take an avid interest in technical equipment and are not satisfied by simplistic explanations of its function! Some patients may however become dependent both mentally and physically on the equipment. An example would be the patient who becomes ventilator dependent after unsuccessful weaning. Watching every move, they become angry and frightened if staff make any alterations to the ventilator settings. It is vital that a bond of trust exists between staff and patient. Settings should not be changed without the patients knowledge and consent as discovery of a change may intensify patient suspicion and distrust.

Many patients learn that the sound of the low pressure alarm, means they are disconnected from the ventilator. Panic reactions may be associated with this, the patient convinced they are unable to breathe without assistance, which may be true.

The methods used to couple the monitoring equipment and

the patient may produce some problems. Adhesive electrodes may affect skin integrity causing irritation and discomfort. Intravascular cannulae and invasive monitoring devices may cause pain, swelling and dysfunction of the limb. Restricted movement adds to patient irritation and discomfort.

Alarm activation and noise created by machine function may cause a good deal of anxiety. False alarms can be distressing and exasperating to patients, relatives and staff. Monotonous noises from machines contributes to the general noise of the environment. The sound of the ventilator may be reassuring to some, but may also cause sensory overload. Some patients may gradually acclimatize to the noise levels, while others find its effects comparable to Chinese water torture.

It can be seen that specialist unit environments have the potential to create intense psychological disturbance. As nurses we must remain aware of the potential adverse consequences of our monitoring care. Adequate explanation, psychological support and anticipation of needs should help make ITU less upsetting for our patients.

GUIDELINES FOR CARE

The patient's spectacles and hearing aid should be available, and if possible a clock and large calender should be within the patient's visual field, for the purpose of orientation in time. Picture charts, pen and paper and nurse call buttons should be within easy reach to facilitate communication.

The nurse should attempt to strike a balance between over and under stimulation of the patient. Adequate sleep and undisturbed rest periods should be permitted, and noise levels should be kept to a minimum. At night the lights should be dimmed, if possible, to give some awareness of day/night and the passage of time.

Relatives should be encouraged to visit often, for short periods. The nursing staff should act as role models, giving advice and guidance on how to be a good and effective visitor. Time can also be used to find out more about the patient and their lifestyle from the visitors. Many people have pet names or preferences, on what they like to be called, it is wise to discover this early. Lack of response to the spoken word may be influenced, if the patient doesn't recognize they are being addressed.

As the patient's condition improves, advice, reassurance and support becomes even more important. The patient should be gently reintroduced to a more normal routine. Persuasion and encouragement act as positive reinforcement of the patient's ability to make more decisions for themselves. For some patients the weaning process from the ITU environment with all its monitoring can be made less traumatic by transfer to a high dependency unit where the ratio of staff to patient is high, but the emphasis on care is more closely allied to self care and increased independence.

Physiologically, as well as psychologically, ITU patients can suffer privation and pain. It should also be remembered that nobody has yet invented an automatic pain monitor. The nearest thing to such a concept is the patient himself and the ITU nurse! Support and help is vital to prevent permanent damage occurring. Adjustment to the stressful environment is often difficult for all concerned. With care and insight nurses can do much to alleviate patient distress and ensure comfort, solace and a sense of security. It is important to explain the equipment and the reasons for its use in words the patient can understand. Many patients may experience a degree of amnesia, forgetting information easily, making repetition necessary. Procedures must be explained before being carried out and it must never be assumed that the patient cannot hear or understand. Conversations about the patient or others should not be held within the patient's hearing range, and medical staff may need reminding that discussion of other cases should be carried out away from the bedside.

RELATIVES IN THE SPECIALIZED UNIT

Relatives of critically ill patients, often arrive at the hospital, sometimes after a long journey, with little idea of what to expect. The patient may appear disfigured and in some cases unrecognizable, from injuries or from the presence of tubes, infusions and other monitoring devices. A relative may arrive alone, and therefore have no support or help from other family members or friends. Relatives are therefore very reliant on information, from hospital staff about the patient's condition and likely prognosis.

Most people find the complex monitoring equipment frightening. They may spend long hours staring at the monitor screens, unsure as to what it shows and apprehensive that the staff might miss some important change. Alarm activation may provoke extreme responses from the relatives. It is even possible that removal of monitoring equipment may be misconstrued as a withdrawal of treatment, leading to hostility and aggression towards the staff member. The nurse must be prepared to be closely watched as he/she performs nursing care. The relatives have ample time to spare and may spend some of it comparing techniques and performance of each nurse.

The nurse has an important function as a role model. Confidence and a caring attitude will help alleviate visitors fears and encourage participation in both the physiological and psychological care of the patient. The visitor after all has nothing to do but watch and endlessly wait. Relatives may ask every member of staff the same questions, hoping that one of them may be optimistic. Honesty when dealing with patients and relatives is vital. If visitors lose trust in staff, the patient's recovery may be affected, the visitor may feel pressurized to stay, to remain anxious and unable to rest.

The presence of monitoring devices may seriously reduce the visitors contact with the patient due to fear of dislodging tubes or infusions etc. The natural reaction at times of stress is to seek physical closeness and be reassured by this contact. In this unnatural situation the relative is inhibited and fearful of touching the patient.

The patient influences and is influenced by their family members. The patient's recovery is often closely linked to the support and the help from their family. It is therefore important to recognize the relatives needs and to give support, guidance and a friendly ear during this stressful time. The relatives feel an intense need to remain close to their loved ones, this should not however be to the exclusion of their own health and welfare. Fatigue, tiredness and boredom are factors which must be understood by hospital staff. Guilt about leaving and fears that if they do leave 'something' might happen should be tactfully and carefully explored and the visitor's decision must be respected.

Most relatives are fearful of being a nuisance, they desperately wish to help in some way and may wish to be involved in the delivery of patient care. A decision by a relative not to help in delivery of care must be seen in this context if it is to be understood by nursing staff. Good levels of communication between relatives and hospital staff maintains good relationships and fosters trust and reassurance. Identification and explanation of monitoring equipment encourages the visitor to relax and feel secure that the patient is safe and that the staff are able and competent.

Helping relatives focus on immediate problems is important, many relatives feel guilty that they were unable to prevent the patient's illness or accident, or they may be worrying unnecessarily about future plans. Assisting in decision making, allowing the relatives to vent their emotions and acknowledging their grief help to reduce their anxieties and maintains their morale.

In the ITU, strong, if sometimes brief, bonds are forged between relatives and staff. Time available to talk to relatives is often short, but it must be used effectively to ensure the relatives receive adequate assistance and support. Care of the relatives is one of the most important aspects of ITU work. Nurses may receive little feedback from their patients, but links with relatives provide the opportunity and challenge for the nurses interpersonal and communication skills.

NURSING STAFF

Sensory overload is not restricted to patients and visitors to the unit. New staff find themselves surrounded by complex and frightening machinery. One of two opposite reactions may occur. The first, is the nurse who fails to see the patient in the bed, only seeing the monitors. The second, is the nurse who fails to see the equipment and concentrates solely on the patient in an attempt to suppress anxiety. Fear that they may be left to cope with the care of a seriously ill patient and with equipment they are not familiar with is a major problem for new ITU staff. Adequate orientation and teaching programmes, allied to support from a mentor, will help new staff adapt to this sometimes difficult nursing specialty. The hazards to the patients, or complex monitoring systems have been discussed earlier. However, the benefits derived from their use are enormous. Invasive monitoring gives important information as to the patient's condition, and permits prompt detection and treatment of potentially life threatening conditions. The patient can be left to rest with minimal disturbance whilst automatic recordings are taken. The nurse must always be aware of the dangers of over reliance on sometimes temperamental equipment and be prepared to double check abnormal readings manually before potentially serious treatment regimes are instituted for non existent conditions. The stress factors within ITU also include the high percentage death rate, dealing with distressed relatives and receiving little feedback from patients. Much of the work is repetitive, in particular taking observations and recording data.

Delegation of workload is important, caring for difficult and demanding patients can be wearing to the morale and the temper! As the nurse will be allocated to one patient for a span of duty, this may cause stress, as the nurse will be unable to leave the patient except for meal breaks etc.

As the nurse's knowledge and confidence in his/her own skills improves then dilemmas posed by treatments ordered by medical staff may conflict with the nurses own values and judgement. The effects of caring for patients whose prognosis seems hopeless are many. Morale may be affected and in some cases conflict of interests and opinions can occur.

General lack of feedback about unit issues, both from superiors and peers can affect the ITU staff morale. Ward meetings, staff development and training programmes, including active encouragement of participation in the day to day running of the unit, will help maintain the cohesiveness of the group and ensure the smooth running of the unit.

A further factor in the stress felt by ITU staff is the rotational night duty shift patterns. Circadian rhythms are affected causing a reduction in performance, minimum performance being attained at around 04.00 hours. In the light of this, it will be recognized that monitoring equipment must have fail safe mechanisms. Alarms indicating serious changes in patient condition must always be used. Observation of monitoring screens becomes boring and tedious. Dysrhythmia's may be unrecognized, undetected or misinterpreted. Patient safety is the prime objective when using monitoring devices.

Monitoring patients is a serious matter as the hazards to the patient are many. Intelligent use of complex monitoring systems however ensures early detection of problems, and prompt instigation of treatment. This permits the patient to rest undisturbed whilst being closely supervised, the ideal situation.

EFFECTS OF MONITORING — EXERCISES

1 What factors may cause the patient to become confused and disorientated?
2 What do you understand by the term Circadian rhythm?
3 What is sensory overload?
4 What may precipitate sensory overload?
5 List the ways in which nurses can prevent the adverse psychological effects experienced by patients?
6 What effects does admission of the patient to hospital have on their relatives?
7 In what ways can a nurse support and assist relatives of patients in specialist units?
8 What factors may lead to stress and low morale in nurses working in ITU?

References

Abels L. (1986). *Critical Care Nursing: A Physiologic Approach.* USA: C. V. Mosby Company.

Asbury A. J. (1985). Patients Memories and Reactions to Intensive Care. *Care of the Critically Ill*, 1, 2.

Atkinson R. S., Hamblin J. J., Wright J. E. C., (1981). *Handbook of Intensive Care.* London: Chapman and Hall Ltd.

Auld Bruya M., Demand J. K. (1985). Nursing Decision Making in Critical Care: Traditional Versus Invasive Blood Pressure Monitoring. *Nursing Administration Quarterly*, Summer 1985.

Bren C., Dracup K. (1978). Helping the spouses of Critically Ill Patients. *American Journal of Nursing*, January, pp. 51–53.

Burgeners S. (1985). Circadian Rhythms: Implications for Evaluation of the Critically Ill Patient. *Critical Care Nurse*, 5, 5.

Carrie L. E. S., Sampson P. J. (1982). *Understanding Anaesthesia.* Oxford: Heinemann Medical Books.

Cohen A. T. (1987). Modes of Ventilation: SIMV For All? *Intensive Care World*, 4, 2, June 1987.

Daley L. (1984). The Perceived Immediate Needs of Families with Relatives in the Intensive Care Setting. *Heart and Lung*, 13, 3, May 1984.

Daly B. J. (1980). Intensive Care Nursing. Second Edition. USA: Medical Examination Publishing Co. Ltd.

Deardon N. M. (1985). Intracranial Pressure Monitoring. *Care of the Critically Ill*, 1, 5, pp. 8–13.

Gardiner J. (1981). *The ECG — What Does It Tell.* Gloucester, England: Stanley Thornes Ltd.

Green J. H. (1976). *An Introduction to Human Physiology.* England: Oxford University Press.

Hampton J. R. (1977). *The ECG Made Easy.* Edinburgh: Churchill Livingstone.

Hawkins L. H., Armstrong E. (1978). Circadian Rhythms and Night Shift Working in Nurses. *Nursing Times*, May 4th, 1978.

Hilgard E. R., Atkinsonrita L., Atkinson R. C. (1977). *Introduction to Psychology*, Seventh Edition. Harcourt Brace Jovanovich Inc.

James P. (1982). Relatively Speaking. *Nursing Mirror*, August 25th, 1982.

Jones-Horner A., Mechsner W. K. (1985). Bedside Insertion of ICP Monitoring Devices. *Critical Care Nurse*, 5, 4, pp. 21–27

Julian D. G. (1978). *Cardiology*, Third Edition. London: Bailliere Tindall Publishers (Cassell Ltd).

King S. L., Gregor F. M. (1985). Stress and Coping in Families of the Critically Ill. *Critical Care Nurse*, 5, 4, pp. 48–51.

Lewis D. J. Robinson J. A. Assessment of Coping Strategies of ICU Nurses in Response to Stress. *Critical Care Nurse*, 6, 6, pp. 38–42.

Lippold O. C. J., Winton F. R. (1979). *Human Physiology*. Edinburgh, London: Churchill Livingstone.

Mackinnon-Kesler S. (1983). Maximising Your ICU Patient's Sensory and Perceptual Environment. *Canadian Nurse*, May 1983, pp. 41–45.

McCulloch J., Townsend A., Williams D. O. (1985). *Focus on Coronary Care*. Oxford: Heinemann Medical Books.

McGhie A. (1979). *Psychology as Applied to Nursing*. Edinburgh, London: Churchill Livingstone.

McNamara, M., Quinn C. (1981). Epidural Intracranial Pressure Monitoring: Theory and Clinical Application. *Journal of Neurosurgical Nursing*, 3, 5, pp. 267–281.

Meltzer I. E., Pinneo R, Kitchell J., Roderick M. D. (1977). *Intensive Coronary Care, A Manual for Nurses*, Third Edition. USA: Charles Press Publishers.

Millar S., Sampson, L. K., Soukup M., Weinberg S. L. (1980). Methods in Critical Care. The AACN Manual. USA: W. B. Saunders Company.

Narwin Hansell H. (1984). The Behavioural Effects of Noise on Man: The Patient with 'Intensive Care Psychosis', *Heart and Lung*, 13, 1, January 1984.

Neutze J. M., Moller C. T., Harris E. A., Horsburgh M. P., Wilson M. D. (1982). *Intensive Care of the Heart and Lungs*, Third Edition. Blackwell Scientific Publications.

Oh T. E. (1981). *Intensive Care Manual*, Second Edition. Sydney, Australia: Butterworths.

Poole-Wilson P. A. (1978). Interpretation of Haemodynamic Measurements. *British Journal of Hospital Medicine*, October 1978.

Resuscitation Council of the United Kingdom (1985). *Cardiopulmonary Resuscitation*.

Ryan D. W. (1982). Morbidity of Intensive Care. *Hospital Update*, October 1982, pp. 1287–96.

Sherwood-Jones E. (1978). *Essential Intensive Care*. England: MTP Press Ltd.

Tinker J., Porter S. W. (1980). A Course in Intensive Therapy Nursing. England: Edward Arnold Ltd.

Woods S. L. (1976). Monitoring Pulmonary Artery Pressures. *American Journal of Nursing*, 76, 11, November 1976.

Index